I0063567

Ultrasound Elastography

Ultrasound Elastography

Special Issue Editor

Christoph F. Dietrich

MDPI • Basel • Beijing • Wuhan • Barcelona • Belgrade

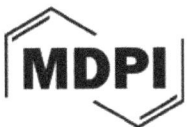

MDPI

Special Issue Editor
Christoph F. Dietrich
Caritas Krankenhaus Bad Mergentheim
Germany

Editorial Office
MDPI
St. Alban-Anlage 66
4052 Basel, Switzerland

This is a reprint of articles from the Special Issue published online in the open access journal *Applied Sciences* (ISSN 2076-3417) from 2017 to 2018 (available at: https://www.mdpi.com/journal/applsci/special_issues/Ultrasound_Elastography).

For citation purposes, cite each article independently as indicated on the article page online and as indicated below:

LastName, A.A.; LastName, B.B.; LastName, C.C. Article Title. *Journal Name* **Year**, *Article Number, Page Range.*

ISBN 978-3-03897-910-4 (Pbk)
ISBN 978-3-03897-911-1 (PDF)

© 2019 by the authors. Articles in this book are Open Access and distributed under the Creative Commons Attribution (CC BY) license, which allows users to download, copy and build upon published articles, as long as the author and publisher are properly credited, which ensures maximum dissemination and a wider impact of our publications.
The book as a whole is distributed by MDPI under the terms and conditions of the Creative Commons license CC BY-NC-ND.

Contents

About the Special Issue Editor

Christoph F. Dietrich, Prof. Dr., MBA, is Chief of Internal Medicine 2 at Caritas-Krankenhaus Bad Mergentheim, Germany. He has also studied philosophy and history. He specializes in internal medicine, gastroenterology, hepatology, proctology, pneumology, hematology, oncology, palliative care, and geriatric medicine. He was the President of EFSUMB from 2013 to 2015 and of DGE-BV in 2013, and he is currently the Vice President of WFUMB (2017–2019).

applied
sciences

MDPI

Editorial

Editorial on the Special Issue of Applied Sciences on the Topic of Elastography

Christoph F. Dietrich [1,2,*] and Jeffrey C. Bamber [3]

1   Sino-German Tongji-Caritas Research Center of Ultrasound in Medicine, Department of Medical Ultrasound, Tongji Hospital, Tongji Medical College, Huazhong University of Science and Technology, Wuhan 430030, China
2   Department of Internal Medicine 2, Medizinische Klinik 2, Caritas Krankenhaus Bad Mergentheim, Uhlandstraße 7, 97980 Bad Mergentheim, Germany
3   Joint Department of Physics and Cancer Research UK Imaging Centre, The Institute of Cancer Research and The Royal Marsden Hospital, Cotswold Road, Sutton, London SM2 5NG, UK; Jeff.Bamber@icr.ac.uk
*   Correspondence: christoph.dietrich@ckbm.de; Tel.: +49-7931-58-2201; Fax: +49-7931-58-2290

Received: 20 June 2018; Accepted: 17 July 2018; Published: 26 July 2018

Keywords: guideline; EFSUMB; WFUMB; elastography; contrast enhanced ultrasound; point of care ultrasound; health care

Elastography is the science of creating noninvasive images of the mechanical characteristics of tissues. The basic principles of elastography have been described some years ago and have remained unchanged since they were outlined in the European Federation of Societies for Ultrasound in Medicine and Biology (EFSUMB) guidelines [1,2]. The first elastography guidelines worldwide were introduced and published by EFSUMB in April 2013 [1,2], were updated in 2017 for the liver [3,4], and were followed by the Japanese Society of Ultrasound in Medicine (JSUM) [5] and the World Federation for Ultrasound in Medicine and Biology (WFUMB) guidelines on basic principles [6] and applications in various organs [7–14]. The mentioned guidelines provide an introduction to the physical principles and technology on which all forms of current commercially available ultrasound elastography are based. The practical advantages and disadvantages that are associated with each of the techniques are described, and guidance is provided on the optimisation of scanning technique, image display, image interpretation, and some of the known image artefacts. The EFSUMB and the WFUMB guideline articles can be freely downloaded from the EFSUMB website (www.efsumb.org) [15] and the WFUMB website (www.wfumb.org).

As described in [1], ultrasound elastography uses ultrasonic echoes to observe tissue displacement as a function of time and space after applying a force that is either dynamic (e.g., by thumping or vibrating) or varying it so slowly that it is considered "quasi-static" (e.g., by probe palpation). The commercially available technologies can be classified according to whether this tissue displacement is (a) displayed directly as the imaged quantity, as in the method that is known as acoustic radiation force impulse (ARFI) imaging; (b) used to calculate and display strain, producing what is termed strain elastography (SE); or (c) used to calculate and display an image of shear wave speed. The last of these is an image that is, in principle, quantitative for a tissue property and is the only one that requires the creation of a shear wave, which in turn requires the use of a dynamic force. The others may use a dynamic force but can also work with a static or nearly static force [1]. However, even the measurement of shear wave speed is dependent on system parameters such as the applied shear force and the frequency of the shear wave. Elastography may be considered as a type of remote palpation that allows the measurement and display of biomechanical properties that are associated with the elastic restoring forces in the tissue that act against shear deformation. This view unifies the different types of elastography, namely SE, ARFI imaging, and SWE, and explains why they all display images with contrast for the same underlying information, which is associated with the shear elastic modulus.

A variety of methods that measure shear wave speed should be grouped under the term shear wave elastography (SWE). These include systems that calculate either the regional values of shear wave speed (without making images) using methods referred to as transient elastography (TE, including vibration-controlled transient elastography, VCTE) and point shear-wave elastography (pSWE), or images of shear wave speed using methods referred to as 2D (or 3D) shear-wave elastography (SWE). The type of elastography that is most suited to the assessment of diffuse liver disease is SWE, which measures the speed of a shear wave in the liver. In the 2017 update of the European guidelines [3,4], VCTE is regarded as a type of SWE, although it differs from other SWE methods because it uses a body-surface vibration to create a shear wave which then travels to the liver, whereas the other methods use acoustic radiation force to create the shear wave within the liver. Recently, normal values of quantities that were measured by SWE of the liver have been summarized [16] and the official American Gastroenterological Association Institute (AGAI) Guidelines on the Role of Elastography in the Evaluation of Liver Fibrosis have been published [17]. Unfortunately, despite the title of the AGAI guidelines paper, it focuses only on the role of VCTE in the evaluation of liver fibrosis, ignoring the fact that the term elastography covers all of the technologies mentioned above. This approach might indicate to the reader that elastography equates only to one commercially available equipment, the Fibroscan®, manufactured only by Echosens, which implements VCTE. This is not true. The review also classifies VCTE as an imaging-based fibrosis assessment, which it is not. VCTE as implemented on the Fibroscan® does not display an anatomical image, although, interestingly, General Electric has recently announced that the Echosens technology has been integrated into its conventional ultrasound system.

Guidelines were introduced in part because of the extremely rapid spread of the use of elastography systems in the clinic once the technology had become commercially available. It is worth mentioning that new methods can be clinically valid and yet are not always (or are rarely) supported by the highest ranking scientific evidence, namely by randomized trials. Often these innovations are so obviously of benefit that randomized controlled trials comparing them with older, less safe or less effective techniques could be deemed unethical.

Elastography can be applied to examine almost all organs in the human body. We refer to a variety of clinical papers with practical applications in the thyroid [9,18–22], pancreas [13], prostate [10,23,24], and endoscopic (endorectal) ultrasound applications [25–27] including the endobronchial use of elastography [28].

The current special issue of Applied Sciences deals with a wide range of elastography methods from many different points of view including open issues of the liver, thyroid, and magnetic resonance elastography (MRE), as well as applications in selected patient groups, e.g., pediatric patients.

MRE is an alternative to ultrasound elastography which has been described in a number of reviews, including [29–31]. The modern method was originated by the Mayo Clinic in 1995 [32] and, like ultrasound elastography, the technique has evolved with a number of technical variations. As with ultrasound elastography, MRE begins by measuring tissue displacement as a function of time and space. Variations exist both in terms of the motion encoding and displacement readout strategies [33] and with respect to algorithms that are used to reconstruct the viscoelastic properties from the measured displacements [34]. As with ultrasound elastography, considerable technical development continues to take place in a research context. One difference to ultrasound elastography is that although quasistatic MRE has long existed (based on a technique known as MR tagging [35]), and it provides cardiac strain assessment [36,37], it is dynamic methods that emerged into widespread clinical use, and 3D-SWE is the ultrasound elastography method that is the closest equivalent of most MRE. However, although acoustic radiation force has been tried as a method of generating displacement, MRE routinely employs harmonic vibrations that are generated by a relatively complex external MR-compatible mechanical device. The clinical use of MRE is less widespread than that of ultrasound elastography, which is likely to be due to a combination of factors, including the high entry-cost, the more limited regulatory approval, the relatively few manufacturers, the relative difficulty of patient set-up, the lack of system portability, and the relatively long examination time. Nevertheless, MRE offers a number of advantages over ultrasound elastography, such as the ability to make elastograms of parts of the body which ultrasound cannot reach (the brain transcranially and the lungs), as well as its intrinsic: controlled-frequency of vibration, 3D imaging, ability to image both elastic and viscous moduli, and capability to provide elastic anisotropy information (i.e., as a function of the direction of shear wave propagation). Commercial ultrasound elastography has yet to evolve some of these technical capabilities which arguably makes current MRE potentially more accurate and precise than current ultrasound elastography. This may explain why recent comparisons suggest that, although ultrasound and MR elastography both have good accuracy for identifying and staging liver fibrosis, MRE is the more accurate of the two [31,38–41]. Nevertheless, they each have technical strengths and limitations; ultrasound elastography may be unreliable in obese patients or where intercostal access is limited, and MRE quality may be poor in patients with substantial iron deposition [41].

The paper on the "Effect of HCV Core Antigen and RNA Clearance during Therapy with Direct Acting Antivirals on Hepatic Stiffness Measured with Shear Wave Elastography in Patients with Chronic Viral Hepatitis" C showed that liver stiffness significantly declined during and after successful antiviral treatment [42]. So far, liver stiffness monitoring during antiviral therapy has been mostly published using TE. Published data on patients who were treated with direct antiviral agents (DAAs) suggest that liver stiffness declines during treatment in patients with advanced fibrosis [43–49]. The decline in liver stiffness reflects more the reduction of inflammatory changes of the liver than it does in true fibrosis.

The paper "Interpretation US Elastography in Chronic Hepatitis B with or without Anti-HBV Therapy" concludes that 2D-SWE (regrettably referred to as ARFI) is a reliable tool for the measurement of liver fibrosis in chronic hepatitis B patients with alanine aminotransferase <5× the upper limit of normal. For those patients under anti-HBV therapy, the optimal timing for SWE analysis will be over 1 to 2.5 years of nucleos(t)ide analogue therapy [50].

The paper "Shear Wave Elastography Combining with Conventional Grey Scale Ultrasound Improves the Diagnostic Accuracy in Differentiating Benign and Malignant Thyroid Nodules" tackles the issue of the differential diagnosis of thyroid nodules. In patients with normal thyroid parenchyma, elastography can rule out malignancy with a high level of certainty if the lesion is displayed as soft. A stiff lesion can be either benign or malignant [51]. The same is true for other parenchymatous organs, e.g., the pancreas [52].

"Non-Invasive Assessment of Hepatic Fibrosis by Elastic Measurement of Liver Using Magnetic Resonance Tagging Images" is a paper that aims to overcome the disadvantage of MRE mentioned above, i.e., that it normally requires an MR-compatible mechanical vibrator which complicates patient set-up. Multiple locations covering a grid in the liver were tracked using MR tagging during liver displacement that was caused by forced exhalation. Two features were then extracted from the resulting time-varying grid patterns, bending energy and the difference between the spatial Fourier transforms of the grid from one moment to another. These features summarize the overall non-rigid deformation in the liver, both normal and shear strain. The more rigid the liver, the lower the values for both of these types of features. In preliminary testing on 17 normal and 17 abnormal liver cases (6 chronic hepatitis cases and 11 liver cirrhosis cases), with manual intervention in setting grid landmarks for tracking, only one abnormal liver was misclassified as normal by a bivariate linear classifier. Although the method does not result in a quantitative tissue property value such as an elastic modulus, its simplicity makes it worthy of further evaluation after development to improve its automated landmark setting.

The paper "Current knowledge in ultrasound based elastography of pediatric patients" reviews the current available literature on the use of SWE in children. Shear wave elastography techniques can be applied in children for the evaluation of liver fibrosis in several etiologies. However, for most pathologies, the evidence is still limited. The confounding factors are similar in adults, including the degree of inflammation and necrosis, iron and copper deposits, cholestasis, and congestions [53].

Funding: For J.C.B. and C.F.D., this research received no external funding.

Conflicts of Interest: J.C.B. declares membership of the advisory board of Supersonic Imagine and Michelson Diagnostics, and collaboration agreements with Phoenix Solutions, Zonare, iThera Medical and Delphinus. C.F.D. declares membership of the advisory board of Hitachi Medical Systems, Siemens Healthineers, Mindray and collaboration agreements with Supersonic Imagine, Olympus and GE. In addition honoraria are also reported for Bracco and Pentax.

References

1. Bamber, J.; Cosgrove, D.; Dietrich, C.F.; Fromageau, J.; Bojunga, J.; Calliada, F.; Cantisani, V.; Correas, J.M.; D'Onofrio, M.; Drakonaki, E.E.; et al. EFSUMB guidelines and recommendations on the clinical use of ultrasound elastography. Part 1: Basic principles and technology. *Ultraschall Med.* **2013**, *34*, 169–184. [CrossRef] [PubMed]

2. Cosgrove, D.; Piscaglia, F.; Bamber, J.; Bojunga, J.; Correas, J.M.; Gilja, O.H.; Klauser, A.S.; Sporea, I.; Calliada, F.; Cantisani, V.; et al. EFSUMB guidelines and recommendations on the clinical use of ultrasound elastography. Part 2: Clinical applications. *Ultraschall Med.* **2013**, *34*, 238–253. [PubMed]

3. Dietrich, C.F.; Bamber, J.; Berzigotti, A.; Bota, S.; Cantisani, V.; Castera, L.; Cosgrove, D.; Ferraioli, G.; Friedrich-Rust, M.; Gilja, O.H.; et al. EFSUMB Guidelines and Recommendations on the Clinical Use of Liver Ultrasound Elastography, Update 2017 (Long Version). *Ultraschall Med.* **2017**, *38*, e16–e47. [CrossRef] [PubMed]

4. Dietrich, C.F.; Bamber, J.; Berzigotti, A.; Bota, S.; Cantisani, V.; Castera, L.; Cosgrove, D.; Ferraioli, G.; Friedrich-Rust, M.; Gilja, O.H.; et al. EFSUMB Guidelines and Recommendations on the Clinical Use of Liver Ultrasound Elastography, Update 2017 (Short Version). *Ultraschall Med.* **2017**, *38*, 377–394. [CrossRef] [PubMed]

5. Shiina, T. JSUM ultrasound elastography practice guidelines: Basics and terminology. *J. Med. Ultrason.* **2013**, *40*, 309–323. [CrossRef] [PubMed]

6. Shiina, T.; Nightingale, K.R.; Palmeri, M.L.; Hall, T.J.; Bamber, J.C.; Barr, R.G.; Castera, L.; Choi, B.I.; Chou, Y.H.; Cosgrove, D.; et al. WFUMB guidelines and recommendations for clinical use of ultrasound elastography: Part 1: Basic principles and terminology. *Ultrasound Med. Biol.* **2015**, *41*, 1126–1147. [CrossRef] [PubMed]

7. Barr, R.G.; Nakashima, K.; Amy, D.; Cosgrove, D.; Farrokh, A.; Schafer, F.; Bamber, J.C.; Castera, L.; Choi, B.I.; Chou, Y.H.; et al. WFUMB guidelines and recommendations for clinical use of ultrasound elastography: Part 2: Breast. *Ultrasound Med. Biol.* **2015**, *41*, 1148–1160. [CrossRef] [PubMed]

8. Ferraioli, G.; Filice, C.; Castera, L.; Choi, B.I.; Sporea, I.; Wilson, S.R.; Cosgrove, D.; Dietrich, C.F.; Amy, D.; Bamber, J.C.; et al. WFUMB guidelines and recommendations for clinical use of ultrasound elastography: Part 3: Liver. *Ultrasound Med. Biol.* **2015**, *41*, 1161–1179. [CrossRef] [PubMed]

9. Cosgrove, D.; Barr, R.; Bojunga, J.; Cantisani, V.; Chammas, M.C.; Dighe, M.; Vinayak, S.; Xu, J.M.; Dietrich, C.F. WFUMB Guidelines and Recommendations on the Clinical Use of Ultrasound Elastography: Part 4. Thyroid. *Ultrasound Med. Biol.* **2017**, *43*, 4–26. [CrossRef] [PubMed]

10. Barr, R.G.; Cosgrove, D.; Brock, M.; Cantisani, V.; Correas, J.M.; Postema, A.W.; Salomon, G.; Tsutsumi, M.; Xu, H.X.; Dietrich, C.F. WFUMB guidelines and recommendations on the clinical use of ultrasound elastography: Part 5. prostate. *Ultrasound Med. Biol.* **2017**, *43*, 27–48. [CrossRef] [PubMed]

11. Kudo, M.; Shiina, T.; Moriyasu, F.; Iijima, H.; Tateishi, R.; Yada, N.; Fujimoto, K.; Morikawa, H.; Hirooka, M.; Sumino, Y.; et al. JSUM ultrasound elastography practice guidelines: Liver. *J. Med. Ultrason.* **2013**, *40*, 325–357. [CrossRef] [PubMed]

12. Nakashima, K.; Shiina, T.; Sakurai, M.; Enokido, K.; Endo, T.; Tsunoda, H.; Takada, E.; Umemoto, T.; Ueno, E. JSUM ultrasound elastography practice guidelines: Breast. *J. Med. Ultrason.* **2013**, *40*, 359–391. [CrossRef] [PubMed]

13. Hirooka, Y.; Kuwahara, T.; Irisawa, A.; Itokawa, F.; Uchida, H.; Sasahira, N.; Kawada, N.; Itoh, Y.; Shiina, T. JSUM ultrasound elastography practice guidelines: Pancreas. *J. Med. Ultrason.* **2015**, *42*, 151–174. [CrossRef] [PubMed]

14. Berzigotti, A.; Ferraioli, G.; Bota, S.; Gilja, O.H.; Dietrich, C.F. Novel ultrasound-based methods to assess liver disease: The game has just begun. *Dig. Liver Dis.* **2018**, *50*, 107–112. [CrossRef] [PubMed]

15. Dietrich, C.F.; Rudd, L.; Saftiou, A.; Gilja, O.H. The EFSUMB website, a great source for ultrasound information and education. *Med. Ultrason.* **2017**, *19*, 102–110. [CrossRef] [PubMed]

16. Dong, Y.; Sirli, R.; Ferraioli, G.; Sporea, I.; Chiorean, L.; Cui, X.; Fan, M.; Wang, W.P.; Gilja, O.H.; Sidhu, P.S.; et al. Shear wave elastography of the liver—Review on normal values. *Z. Gastroenterol.* **2017**, *55*, 153–166. [CrossRef] [PubMed]

17. Lim, J.K.; Flamm, S.L.; Singh, S.; Falck-Ytter, Y.T. Clinical Guidelines Committee of the American Gastroenterological, A American Gastroenterological Association Institute Guideline on the Role of Elastography in the Evaluation of Liver Fibrosis. *Gastroenterology* **2017**, *152*, 1536–1543. [CrossRef] [PubMed]

18. Dighe, M.; Barr, R.; Bojunga, J.; Cantisani, V.; Chammas, M.C.; Cosgrove, D.; Cui, X.W.; Dong, Y.; Fenner, F.; Radzina, M.; et al. Thyroid Ultrasound: State of the Art Part 1—Thyroid Ultrasound reporting and Diffuse Thyroid Diseases. *Med. Ultrason.* **2017**, *19*, 79–93. [CrossRef] [PubMed]

19. Dighe, M.; Barr, R.; Bojunga, J.; Cantisani, V.; Chammas, M.C.; Cosgrove, D.; Cui, X.W.; Dong, Y.; Fenner, F.; Radzina, M.; et al. Thyroid ultrasound: State of the art. part 2—Focal thyroid lesions. *Med. Ultrason.* **2017**, *19*, 195–210. [CrossRef] [PubMed]

20. Friedrich-Rust, M.; Vorlaender, C.; Dietrich, C.F.; Kratzer, W.; Blank, W.; Schuler, A.; Broja, N.; Cui, X.W.; Herrmann, E.; Bojunga, J. Evaluation of strain elastography for differentiation of thyroid nodules: Results of a prospective degum multicenter study. *Ultraschall Med.* **2016**, *37*, 262–270. [CrossRef] [PubMed]

21. Cantisani, V.; Lodise, P.; Di Rocco, G.; Grazhdani, H.; Giannotti, D.; Patrizi, G.; Medvedyeva, E.; Olive, M.; Fioravanti, C.; Giacomelli, L.; et al. Diagnostic accuracy and interobserver agreement of Quasistatic Ultrasound Elastography in the diagnosis of thyroid nodules. *Ultraschall Med.* **2015**, *36*, 162–167. [CrossRef] [PubMed]

22. Grazhdani, H.; Cantisani, V.; Lodise, P.; Di Rocco, G.; Proietto, M.C.; Fioravanti, E.; Rubini, A.; Redler, A. Prospective evaluation of acoustic radiation force impulse technology in the differentiation of thyroid nodules: Accuracy and interobserver variability assessment. *J. Ultrasound* **2014**, *17*, 13–20. [CrossRef] [PubMed]

23. Correas, J.M.; Tissier, A.M.; Khairoune, A.; Vassiliu, V.; Mejean, A.; Helenon, O.; Memo, R.; Barr, R.G. Prostate cancer: Diagnostic performance of real-time shear-wave elastography. *Radiology* **2015**, *275*, 280–289. [CrossRef] [PubMed]

24. Correas, J.M.; Tissier, A.M.; Khairoune, A.; Khoury, G.; Eiss, D.; Helenon, O. Ultrasound elastography of the prostate: State of the art. *Diagn. Interv. Imaging* **2013**, *94*, 551–560. [CrossRef] [PubMed]

25. Dietrich, C.F.; Bibby, E.; Jenssen, C.; Saftoiu, A.; Iglesias-Garcia, J.; Havre, R.F. EUS elastography: How to do it? *Endosc. Ultrasound* **2018**, *7*, 20–28. [CrossRef] [PubMed]

26. Dietrich, C.F.; Barr, R.G.; Farrokh, A.; Dighe, M.; Hocke, M.; Jenssen, C.; Dong, Y.; Saftoiu, A.; Havre, R.F. Strain Elastography—How To Do It? *Ultrasound Int. Open* **2017**, *3*, E137–E149. [CrossRef] [PubMed]

27. Hocke, M.; Braden, B.; Jenssen, C.; Dietrich, C.F. Present status and perspectives of endosonography 2017 in gastroenterology. *Korean J. Int. Med.* **2018**, *33*, 36–63. [CrossRef] [PubMed]

28. Dietrich, C.F.; Jenssen, C.; Herth, F.J. Endobronchial ultrasound elastography. *Endosc. Ultrasound* **2016**, *5*, 233–238. [CrossRef] [PubMed]

29. Mariappan, Y.K.; Glaser, K.J.; Ehman, R.L. Magnetic resonance elastography: A review. *Clin. Anat.* **2010**, *23*, 497–511. [CrossRef] [PubMed]

30. Litwiller, D.V.; Mariappan, Y.K.; Ehman, R.L. Magnetic resonance elastography. *Curr. Med. Imaging Rev.* **2012**, *8*, 46–55. [CrossRef] [PubMed]

31. Low, G.; Kruse, S.A.; Lomas, D.J. General review of magnetic resonance elastography. *World J. Radiol.* **2016**, *8*, 59–72. [CrossRef] [PubMed]

32. Muthupillai, R.; Lomas, D.J.; Rossman, P.J.; Greenleaf, J.F.; Manduca, A.; Ehman, R.L. Magnetic resonance elastography by direct visualization of propagating acoustic strain waves. *Science* **1995**, *269*, 1854–1857. [CrossRef] [PubMed]

33. Guenthner, C.; Kozerke, S. Encoding and readout strategies in magnetic resonance elastography. *NMR Biomed.* **2018**, e3919. [CrossRef] [PubMed]

34. Fovargue, D.; Nordsletten, D.; Sinkus, R. Stiffness reconstruction methods for MR elastography. *NMR Biomed.* **2018**, e3935. [CrossRef] [PubMed]

35. Zerhouni, E.A.; Parish, D.M.; Rogers, W.J.; Yang, A.; Shapiro, E.P. Human heart: Tagging with MR imaging–a method for noninvasive assessment of myocardial motion. *Radiology* **1988**, *169*, 59–63. [CrossRef] [PubMed]

36. Moore, C.C.; O'Dell, W.G.; McVeigh, E.R.; Zerhouni, E.A. Calculation of three-dimensional left ventricular strains from biplanar tagged MR images. *J. Magn. Reson. Imaging* **1992**, *2*, 165–175. [CrossRef] [PubMed]
37. Khan, S.; Fakhouri, F.; Majeed, W.; Kolipaka, A. Cardiovascular magnetic resonance elastography: A review. *NMR Biomed.* **2017**. [CrossRef]
38. Kennedy, P.; Wagner, M.; Castera, L.; Hong, C.W.; Johnson, C.L.; Sirlin, C.B.; Taouli, B. Quantitative elastography methods in liver disease: Current evidence and future directions. *Radiology* **2018**, *286*, 738–763. [CrossRef] [PubMed]
39. Hsu, C.; Caussy, C.; Imajo, K.; Chen, J.; Singh, S.; Kaulback, K.; Le, M.D.; Hooker, J.; Tu, X.; Bettencourt, R.; et al. Magnetic resonance vs. transient elastography analysis of patients with non-alcoholic fatty liver disease: A systematic review and pooled analysis of individual participants. *Clin. Gastroenterol. Hepatol.* **2018**. [CrossRef] [PubMed]
40. Park, C.C.; Nguyen, P.; Hernandez, C.; Bettencourt, R.; Ramirez, K.; Fortney, L.; Hooker, J.; Sy, E.; Savides, M.T.; Alquiraish, M.H.; et al. Magnetic resonance elastography vs. transient elastography in detection of fibrosis and noninvasive measurement of steatosis in patients with biopsy-proven nonalcoholic fatty liver disease. *Gastroenterology* **2017**, *152*, 598–607. [CrossRef] [PubMed]
41. Tang, A.; Cloutier, G.; Szeverenyi, N.M.; Sirlin, C.B. Ultrasound elastography and mr elastography for assessing liver fibrosis: Part 1, principles and techniques. *Am. J. Roentgenol.* **2015**, *205*, 22–32. [CrossRef] [PubMed]
42. Lucejko, M.; Flisiak, R. Effect of HCV core antigen and RNA clearance during therapy with direct acting antivirals on hepatic stiffness measured with shear wave elastography in patients with chronic viral hepatitis C. *Appl. Sci.* **2018**, *8*, 198. [CrossRef]
43. Chan, J.; Gogela, N.; Zheng, H.; Lammert, S.; Ajayi, T.; Fricker, Z.; Kim, A.Y.; Robbins, G.K.; Chung, R.T. Direct-acting antiviral therapy for chronic HCV infection results in liver stiffness regression over 12 months post-treatment. *Digest. Dis. Sci.* **2017**. [CrossRef] [PubMed]
44. Knop, V.; Hoppe, D.; Welzel, T.; Vermehren, J.; Herrmann, E.; Vermehren, A.; Friedrich-Rust, M.; Sarrazin, C.; Zeuzem, S.; Welker, M.W. Regression of fibrosis and portal hypertension in HCV-associated cirrhosis and sustained virologic response after interferon-free antiviral therapy. *J. Viral Hepat.* **2016**, *23*, 994–1002. [CrossRef] [PubMed]
45. Facciorusso, A.; Del Prete, V.; Turco, A.; Buccino, R.V.; Nacchiero, M.C.; Muscatiello, N. Long-term liver stiffness assessment in HCV patients undergoing antiviral therapy: Results from a 5-year cohort study. *J. Gastroenterol. Hepatol.* **2017**, *33*, 942–949. [CrossRef] [PubMed]
46. Ogasawara, N.; Kobayashi, M.; Akuta, N.; Kominami, Y.; Fujiyama, S.; Kawamura, Y.; Sezaki, H.; Hosaka, T.; Suzuki, F.; Saitoh, S.; et al. Serial changes in liver stiffness and controlled attenuation parameter following direct-acting antiviral therapy against hepatitis C virus genotype 1b. *J. Med. Virol.* **2017**, *90*, 313–319. [CrossRef] [PubMed]
47. Persico, M.; Rosato, V.; Aglitti, A.; Precone, D.; Corrado, M.; De Luna, A.; Morisco, F.; Camera, S.; Federico, A.; Dallio, M.; et al. Sustained virological response by direct antiviral agents in HCV leads to an early and significant improvement of liver fibrosis. *Antivir. Ther.* **2017**, *23*, 129–138. [CrossRef] [PubMed]
48. Pons, M.; Santos, B.; Simon-Talero, M.; Ventura-Cots, M.; Riveiro-Barciela, M.; Esteban, R.; Augustin, S.; Genesca, J. Rapid liver and spleen stiffness improvement in compensated advanced chronic liver disease patients treated with oral antivirals. *Ther. Adv. Gastroenterol.* **2017**, *10*, 619–629. [CrossRef] [PubMed]
49. Sporea, I.; Lupusoru, R.; Mare, R.; Popescu, A.; Gheorghe, L.; Iacob, S.; Sirli, R. Dynamics of liver stiffness values by means of transient elastography in patients with HCV liver cirrhosis undergoing interferon free treatment. *J. Gastrointest. Liver Dis.* **2017**, *26*, 145–150. [CrossRef]
50. Lee, C.; Wan, Y.; Hsu, T.; Huang, S.; Yu, M.; Lee, W.; Tsui, P.; Chen, Y.; Lin, C.; Tai, D. Interpretation US elastography in chronic hepatitis B with or without anti-HBV therapy. *Appl. Sci.* **2017**, *7*, 1164. [CrossRef]
51. Baig, F.N.; Liu, S.Y.W.; Lam, H.; Yip, S.; Law, H.K.W.; Ying, M. Shear wave elastography combining with conventional grey scale ultrasound improves the diagnostic accuracy in differentiating benign and malignant thyroid nodules. *Appl. Sci.* **2017**, *7*, 1103. [CrossRef]

52. Ignee, A.; Jenssen, C.; Arcidiacono, P.G.; Hocke, M.; Moller, K.; Saftoiu, A.; Will, U.; Fusaroli, P.; Iglesias-Garcia, J.; Ponnudurai, R.; et al. Endoscopic ultrasound elastography of small solid pancreatic lesions: A multicenter study. *Endoscopy* **2018**. [CrossRef] [PubMed]
53. Dietrich, C.F.; Sirli, R.; Ferraioli, G.; Popescu, A.; Sporea, I.; Pienar, C.; Kunze, C.; Taut, H.; Schrading, S.; Bota, S.; Schreiber-Dietrich, D.; Yi, D. Current Knowledge in Ultrasound-Based Liver Elastography of Pediatric Patients. *Appl. Sci.* **2018**, *8*, 944. [CrossRef]

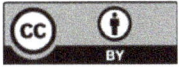

© 2018 by the authors. Licensee MDPI, Basel, Switzerland. This article is an open access article distributed under the terms and conditions of the Creative Commons Attribution (CC BY) license (http://creativecommons.org/licenses/by/4.0/).

applied
sciences

MDPI

Article

Shear Wave Elastography Combining with Conventional Grey Scale Ultrasound Improves the Diagnostic Accuracy in Differentiating Benign and Malignant Thyroid Nodules

Faisal N. Baig [1] , Shirley Y. W. Liu [2], Hoi-Chun Lam [1], Shea-Ping Yip [1] , Helen K. W. Law [1,*] and Michael Ying [1,*]

[1] Department of Health Technology and Informatics, The Hong Kong Polytechnic University, Hung Hom, Kowloon, Hong Kong, China; faisal.baig@connect.polyu.hk (F.N.B.); hoi-chun-eric.lam@connect.polyu.hk (H.-C.L.); shea.ping.yip@polyu.edu.hk (S.-P.Y.)

[2] Department of Surgery, Prince of Wales Hospital, The Chinese University of Hong Kong, Shatin, New Territories, Hong Kong, China; liuyw@surgery.cuhk.edu.hk

* Correspondence: helen.law@polyu.edu.hk (H.K.W.L.); htmying@polyu.edu.hk (M.Y.); Tel.: +86-(852)-3400-8562 (H.K.W.L.); +86-(852)-3400-8566 (M.Y.); Fax: +86-(852)-2362-4365 (H.K.W.L. & M.Y.)

Received: 11 September 2017; Accepted: 13 October 2017; Published: 25 October 2017

Abstract: Shear wave elastography provides information about the stiffness of thyroid nodules that could be a new indicator of malignancy. The current study aimed to investigate the feasibility of using shear wave elastography (SWE) alone and in conjunction with grey scale ultrasound (GSU) to predict malignancy in 111 solitary thyroid nodules. Malignant thyroid nodules tended to have microcalcification, hypoechogenicity, tall to width ratio >1, and irregular borders ($p < 0.05$). SWE indices ($E_{maximum}$ and E_{mean}) of malignant nodules (median $\pm$ standard error: 85.2 $\pm$ 8.1 kPa and 26.6 $\pm$ 2.5 kPa) were significantly higher than those of benign nodules (median $\pm$ standard error: 50.3 $\pm$ 3.1 kPa and 20.2 $\pm$ 1 kPa) ($p < 0.05$). The optimal cut-off of $E_{maximum}$ and E_{mean} for distinguishing benign and malignant nodules was 67.3 kPa and 23.1 kPa, respectively. Diagnostic performances for GSU + $E_{maximum}$, GSU + E_{mean}, GSU, $E_{maximum}$ and E_{mean} were: 70.4%, 74.1%, 96.3%, 70.4% and 74.1% for sensitivity, 83.3%, 79.8%, 46.4%, 70.2%, and 66.7% for specificity, and 80.2%, 78.4%, 58.5%, 70.3%, and 68.5% for accuracy, respectively. Our results suggested that combining GSU with SWE (using $E_{maximum}$ or E_{mean}) increased the overall diagnostic accuracy in distinguishing benign and malignant thyroid nodules.

Keywords: ultrasound; thyroid cancer; shear wave elastography

1. Introduction

Grey scale ultrasound (GSU) is the first-line imaging investigation for the assessment of thyroid nodules [1,2]. Although certain GSU features have been reported to be associated with thyroid malignancy (microcalcification, hypoechogenicity, irregular shape, tall to width ratio >1, absent halo sign, and irregular margins) [3–5], these features may also be found in benign nodules [6,7]. To date, none of the GSU features are known to exhibit a high sensitivity and specificity in differentiating benign and malignant thyroid nodules [8–10].

Fine-needle aspiration cytology (FNAC) is recommended by the American Thyroid Association to evaluate thyroid nodules when the GSU findings are inconclusive [11]. However, potential sampling and analytical errors limit its application in establishing correct diagnosis in some cases such as small thyroid nodules [12,13]. Only about 65–75% of thyroid nodules can be correctly diagnosed by FNAC [14], whilst the remaining 25–35% of nodules yield indeterminate pathology or non-diagnostic results [15]. Both GSU and FNAC have wide ranges of sensitivity (52–97% and 54–90%, respectively), and specificity (26–83% and 60–98%, respectively) in distinguishing benign and malignant thyroid nodules [10,16].

Power Doppler and color Doppler ultrasound evaluate the vascularity of thyroid nodules. It is generally believed that hypervascularity is a feature of thyroid malignancy [17,18]. Some other studies suggested that vascular pattern of thyroid nodules can be useful to predict the thyroid malignancy e.g., thyroid nodules with dominant central vascularity are frequently associated with malignant thyroid nodules, whereas benign thyroid nodules tend to have peripheral vascularity or appear avascular [19,20]. Ultrasound elastography is a non-invasive imaging technique that measures tissue stiffness and provides color-coded elasticity map. In strain elastography (SE), the elasticity color map and strain ratio (SR) provide qualitative and semi-quantitative estimates of elasticity distribution, respectively. SE has limited clinical value due to the need of subjective interpretation of elastogram and compressive maneuvers. Contrarily, shear wave elastography (SWE) is less operator-dependent and more reproducible than SE, and it provides quantitative assessment in the form of elasticity indices ($E_{maximum}$, E_{mean}, $E_{minimum}$). SWE uses focused ultrasound impulses at varying depths in tissue to induce tissue displacement and results in the generation of shear waves which propagate laterally [21]. Shear waves travel faster in harder medium than in softer counterpart, and their velocity is directly proportional to the square root of Young's modulus. Young's modulus measures the tissue stiffness by demonstrating the relationship between stress (applied force) and strain (resultant deformation) [22,23]. Stiffer tissues exhibit higher Young's modulus as compared to softer tissues. In the current study, a higher Young's modulus for malignant nodules (85.2 ± 8.1 kPa) than benign nodule (50.3 ± 3.1 kPa) is observed ($p < 0.05$). Assuming the tissue density 1 g/cm^3, the Poisson's ratio was 0.5 [24,25]. The propagation speed of shear waves is tracked by the ultrafast sonographic tracking technique [26]. By evaluating the speed of shear waves in the tissue, the tissue stiffness can be determined. In comparison to the normal thyroid parenchyma, most malignant thyroid nodules have firm stroma due to the presence of excessive collagen, excessive myofibroblast, and desmoplastic transformation, hence resisting tissue strain upon stress [10,27,28]. Therefore, most of the malignant thyroid nodules tend to be stiffer. As the stiffness of thyroid nodules can be evaluated with shear wave elastography, malignant thyroid nodules tend to have higher shear wave elastography index. In the current study, we hypothesize that malignant thyroid nodules are stiffer than benign nodules on SWE. The present study aimed to evaluate the diagnostic accuracy of SWE in differentiating benign and malignant thyroid nodules when it was used alone and combined with GSU. Positive study results will have implications in the identification of thyroid nodules that need to be further evaluated by FNAC/biopsy, and thus a correct diagnosis can be established.

2. Materials and Methods

2.1. Subject Recruitment

This prospective study was approved by the Human Subject Ethics Sub-committee (HSESC), the Hong Kong Polytechnic University, Hong Kong, and Institutional Review Board of Prince of Wales Hospital, Hong Kong. Informed written consent for the study was obtained from all of the human subjects in accordance with the WORLD Medical Association Declaration of Helsinki: Ethical principles for medical research involving human subjects, 2008 (http://www.wma.net/en/30publications/ 10policies/b3/). The privacy rights of the human subjects in the study were observed.

Between September 2013 and June 2015, a total of 122 consecutive patients (22 men and 100 women, mean age: 53 ± 13.7 years; age range 21–95 years) with 163 thyroid nodules were recruited at the Prince of Wales Hospital, Hong Kong. We included patients who had at least one thyroid nodule diagnosed clinically or radiologically on thyroid ultrasound examination. Exclusion criteria were completely cystic nodules or any forms of inflammatory thyroid diseases (acute thyroiditis, chronic thyroiditis, grave's disease, and sub-acute thyroiditis), which were associated with increased thyroid parenchymal stiffness.

2.2. Ultrasound Examination of Thyroid Gland

GSU and SWE examinations of thyroid gland were performed on both sides of the neck of all patients. Due to the ethical issues and restricted policies of our institution, we had limited data access to the patient's clinical reports. Therefore, we could not check the stage of tumors of the patients. However, we had accessed to the histopathology and fine needle aspiration cytology results for the final diagnosis of the nodules. Cytopathology and/or histopathology diagnoses were used to correlate the accuracy of GSU and SWE findings. All of the thyroid ultrasound examinations were conducted by the same operator (M.Y.) using the same ultrasound unit in conjunction with a 4–15 MHz linear transducer (Aixplorer, Supersonic Imagine, Aix-en-Provence, France). All of the ultrasound examinations were performed with an imaging mechanical index (MI) of 1.5 and the MI of the "push" pulses for the SWE was 1.2. In the thyroid ultrasound examinations, we used a broadband frequency ultrasound transducer, which allows operators to choose different frequencies for examination. In the current study, we standardized the scanning protocol of using high frequency (~15 MHz) to optimize the image quality. During the ultrasound examination, patients were asked to lie in supine position on the examination couch with the neck and shoulders supported by pillow to keep patient's neck slightly hyperextended. A generous amount of coupling gel was applied and GSU was performed to identify any nodule in the thyroid lobes and isthmus. When a thyroid nodule was identified (based on perceived contrast between the echogenicity of thyroid nodule and adjacent thyroid parenchyma), multiple transverse, and longitudinal sonograms of the nodule were obtained. Each nodule was assessed for suspicious grey scale sonographic features [1,21,29,30] including absent halo sign, microcalcification, hypoechogenicity, internal solid echotexture, tall to width ratio >1, and irregular margins (Figures 1 and 2).

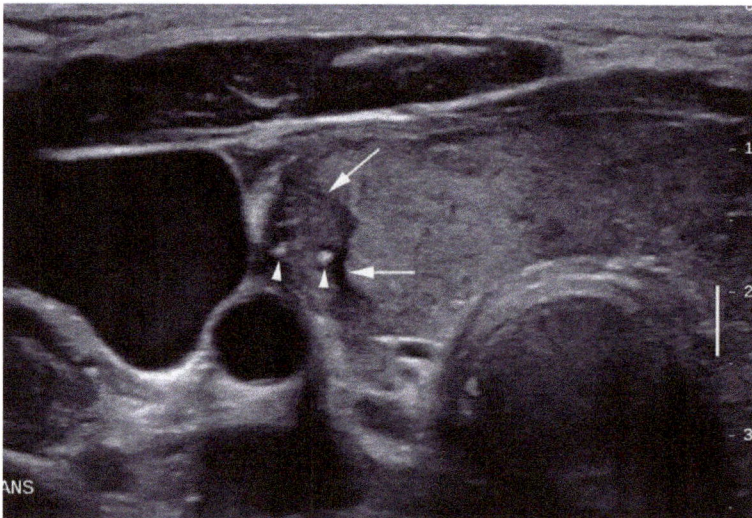

Figure 1. Transverse sonogram showing a papillary carcinoma in the right thyroid lobe of a 43-year-old patient (**arrows**). The tumor is hypoechoic when compare to the adjacent thyroid parenchyma, and has multiple microcalcifications (**arrowheads**).

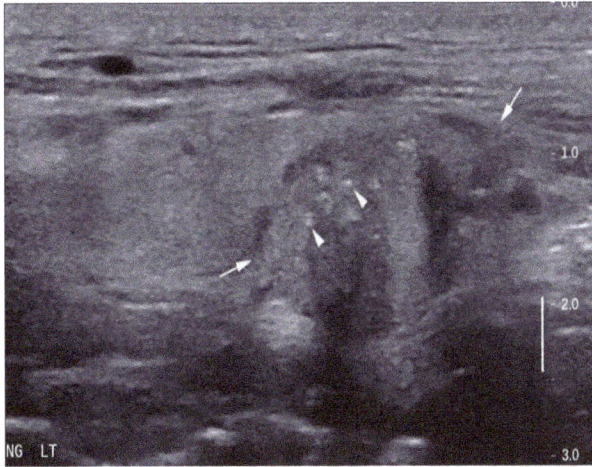

Figure 2. Longitudinal sonogram showing a papillary carcinoma in the left thyroid lobe of a 51-year-old patient (**arrows**). The nodule appeared hypoechoic, ill-defined, and had multiple microcalcifications (**arrowheads**).

After GSU, SWE was then performed on the thyroid nodule. For patients with multiple thyroid nodules, SWE was performed on the largest thyroid nodule, and/or the nodule with one or more suspicious grey scale sonographic features, as described above. In the SWE examination, the size of the SWE acquisition box was first adjusted to cover the entire thyroid nodule. Multiple transverse and longitudinal shear wave elastograms of the nodule were obtained (Figures 3 and 4).

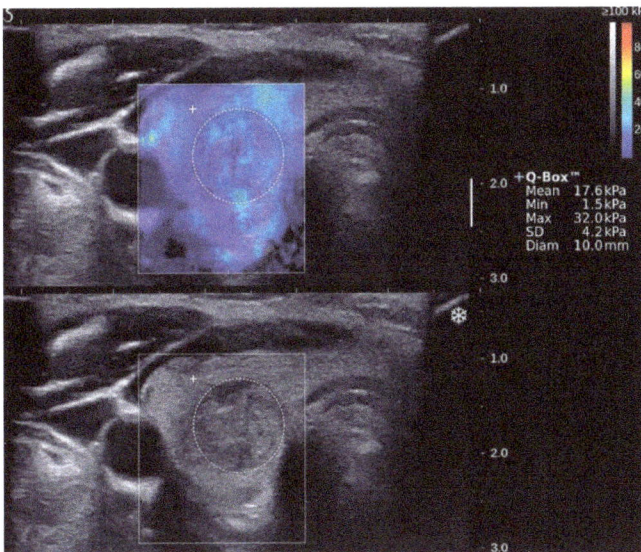

Figure 3. Transverse elastogram (**upper**) and grey scale sonogram (**lower**) of a benign nodule in the right thyroid lobe of a 37-year-old patient. The value of elasticity indices ($E_{maximum}$ = 32 kPa and E_{mean} = 17.6 kPa) were lower than the respective cut-off values reported in the present study.

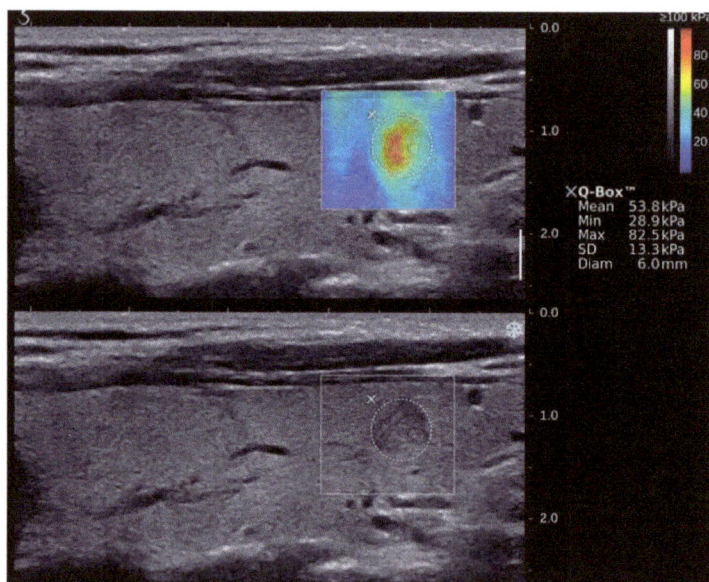

Figure 4. Longitudinal elastogram (**upper**) and grey scale sonogram (**lower**) of a papillary carcinoma in the right thyroid lobe of a 57-year-old patient. The value of elasticity indices ($E_{maximum}$ = 82.5 kPa and E_{mean} = 53.8 kPa) were higher than the respective cut-off values reported in the present study.

To acquire an elastogram, the transducer was held at the same position for at least 2 s to allow the SWE signal acquisition to settle and to reduce variability. During SWE examination, caution was made to avoid compression applying on the patient's neck by the transducer, which might affect the stiffness measurement of thyroid nodules. Taking shear wave elastograms in the scan planes showing calcification within the nodule were avoided. After the ultrasound examination, FNAC was performed on the targeted nodules. Nodules with confirmed malignancy (papillary carcinoma, follicular carcinoma, or medullary carcinoma) or indeterminate cytology (follicular neoplasm, follicular lesion of undetermined significance, atypia of undetermined significance, or repeated non-diagnostic cytology) were further evaluated by surgical resection and histopathological examination.

Before the commencement of the main study, two independent observers (F.N.B. and H.C.L.) conducted an inter-observer reliability test on 50 archived data sets of randomly selected thyroid nodules to evaluate the inter-observer reliability in SWE measurement. The results showed that there was a high inter-observer reliability between the two observers (intraclass correlation coefficient = 0.98). In the current study, archived grey scale sonograms and elastograms were reviewed by single observer who was blinded to the cytology and histology results. Each thyroid nodule was assessed for the presence or absence of suspicious grey scale sonographic features: absent halo sign, microcalcification, hypoechogenicity, internal solid echotexture, tall to width ratio >1, and irregular margins. The hypoechogenicity of thyroid nodules was determined by observer's visual assessment based on the perceived contrast between thyroid nodule and adjacent thyroid parenchyma.

The stiffness of the thyroid nodule was measured using the inbuilt quantification tool of the ultrasound unit (Q-box^{TM}, Supersonic Imagine, Aix-en-Provence, France) on the elastograms. The circular quantification region of interest (ROI) was used to cover the entire thyroid nodule without including the adjacent thyroid parenchyma. The software then automatically calculated the SWE indices ($E_{maximum}$, E_{mean}, and $E_{minimum}$), which were expressed in kilo-pascals (kPa) (Figures 3 and 4). The range of stiffness measurement ranged from 0 kPa to ≥100 kPa. For each thyroid nodule, five measurements with the highest stiffness values were selected from both longitudinal and transverse elastograms, and the average of them was calculated to deduce the mean of $E_{maximum}$, E_{mean} and $E_{minimum}$.

2.3. Data Analysis

Chi square test was used to determine the significance of difference of GSU features between benign and malignant nodules, whereas the significance of difference of SWE indices between benign and malignant nodules was calculated by Mann Whitney U test. The diagnostic performance of GSU was evaluated by deducing the frequency tables of true-positive, true-negative, false-positive, and false-negative cases. Receiver operating characteristic (ROC) curves were used to determine the optimal cut-off of different SWE indices in distinguishing benign and malignant nodules, and the associated diagnostic performance of the optimal cut-off. The diagnostic performance of combining GSU and SWE was determined based on the principle that a thyroid nodule was considered malignant when it was presented with at least one suspicious GSU feature (i.e., hypoechogenicity, tall to width ratio ≥ 1, irregular border or microcalcification) and had SWE indices ($E_{maximum} \geq 67.3$ kPa or $E_{mean} \geq 23.1$ kPa) equal to or greater than the corresponding optimal cut-off values. Thyroid nodules did not fulfill these criteria were categorized as benign. All statistical analyses were performed using the Statistical Package for the Social Sciences (SPSS) software (Version 20, IBM Corporation, Armonk, NY, USA) and two-tailed p value < 0.05 was significant.

3. Results

3.1. Histology Results

In the 122 thyroid nodules evaluated, 73 nodules were confirmed as benign on FNAC. In the remaining 49 nodules, histopathological examination upon surgical resection confirmed 27 nodules to be malignant and 11 benign. The remaining 11 nodules were excluded from the study because surgical resection had not been performed and the final diagnosis could not be obtained. Therefore, altogether, 111 thyroid nodules (27 malignant and 84 benign) were included in this study. Amongst the 27 malignant nodules, there were 23 papillary thyroid carcinomas, 3 follicular thyroid carcinomas and 1 Hurthle cell carcinoma.

3.2. Grey Scale Ultrasound

The grey scale sonographic features of thyroid nodules are summarized in Table 1. Among different grey scale sonographic features, microcalcification (77.8% and 7.1%, respectively), tall to width ratio >1 (59.3% and 13.1%, respectively), hypoechogenicity (92.6% and 33.3%, respectively) and irregular margin (55.6% and 16.7% respectively), were significantly more common in malignant nodules than benign nodules (all $p < 0.05$). There was no significant difference in the absent halo sign and internal solid echotexture between malignant and benign nodules ($p > 0.05$).

With the above results, further data analysis was performed to determine the diagnostic performance of GSU in distinguishing benign and malignant thyroid nodules. In the data analysis, thyroid nodules with at least one of the above four significant grey scale sonographic features (i.e., microcalcification, tall to width ratio >1, hypoechogenicity and irregular margin) were malignant, whereas others were benign. Using these assessment criteria, 26 malignant nodules and 39 benign nodes were correctly identified. Results showed that the sensitivity, specificity, positive predictive value (PPV), negative predictive value (NPV), and overall accuracy of GSU in distinguishing benign and malignant nodules were 96.3%, 46.4%, 36.6%, 97.5% and 58.5% respectively (Table 2).

Table 1. Grey scale sonographic features of benign and malignant thyroid nodules.

Grey Scale Ultrasound Features	Number of Nodules (Percentage)		p-Value (95% Confidence Interval)
	Benign (n = 84)	Malignant (n = 27)	
Microcalcification			
Yes	6 (7.1%)	21 (77.8%)	<0.05
No	78 (92.9%)	6 (22.2%)	(0.12–0.49)
Tall/width ratio >1			
Yes	11 (13.1%)	16 (59.3%)	<0.05
No	73 (86.9%)	11 (40.7%)	(0.29–0.74)
Hypoechogenicity	-	-	-
Yes	28 (33.3%)	25 (92.6%)	<0.05
No	56 (66.7%)	2 (7.4%)	(0.42–0.71)
Irregular margins			
Yes	14 (16.7%)	15 (55.6%)	<0.05
No	70 (83.3%)	12 (44.4%)	(0.38–0.83)
Absent Halo sign			
Yes	74 (88.1%)	26 (96.3%)	>0.05
No	10 (11.9%)	1 (3.7%)	(0.65–1.01)
Internal solid echotexture			
Yes	61 (72.6%)	27 (100%)	>0.05
No	23 (27.4%)	0 (0%)	(0.6–0.8)

Table 2. Diagnostic performance of grey scale ultrasound (GSU), shear wave elastography (SWE) indices and combination of GSU and SWE in evaluation of thyroid nodules.

Ultrasound Techniques	Sensitivity (%)	Specificity (%)	PPV (%)	NPV (%)	Accuracy (%)	AUC
GSU	96.3	46.4	36.6	97.5	58.5	0.714
E_{max} (67.3 kPa)	70.4	70.2	43.2	88.1	70.3	0.785
E_{mean} (23.1 kPa)	74.1	66.7	41.7	88.9	68.5	0.710
GSU + E_{max} (67.3 kPa)	70.4	83.3	57.6	89.7	80.2	0.769
GSU + E_{mean} (23.1 kPa)	74.1	79.8	54.1	90.5	78.4	0.775

GSU, grey scale ultrasound, PPV, positive predictive value; NPV, negative predictive value, AUC, area under the curve.

3.3. Shear Wave Elastography

Table 3 shows the SWE indices of benign and malignant thyroid nodules. The results showed that malignant thyroid nodules were associated with higher SWE indices. The median of $E_{maximum}$ of malignant nodules (85.2 ± 8.1 kPa) was significantly higher than that of benign nodules (50.3 ± 3.1 kPa) ($p < 0.05$). Similarly, the median of E_{mean} of malignant nodules was 26.6 ± 2.5 kPa and of benign nodules was 20.2 ± 1 kPa, and the difference was statistically significant ($p < 0.05$). However, no significant difference was found in $E_{minimum}$ between benign and malignant nodules ($p > 0.05$).

Table 3. Shear wave elastography measurement of benign and malignant thyroid nodules.

SWE Indices	Median ± 1 Standard Error		p-Value (95% Confidence Interval)
	Benign	Malignant	
E_{max}	50.3 ± 3.1	85.2 ± 8.1	<0.05 (50.9–63.5; 73.0–106.1)
E_{mean}	20.2 ± 1.0	26.6 ± 2.5	<0.05 (19.5–23.5; 23.5–33.9)
E_{min}	3.9 ± 0.6	3.8 ± 1.2	>0.05 (4.2–6.4; 3.7–8.8)

Since significant difference was found between benign and malignant nodules in $E_{maximum}$ and E_{mean} only, the evaluation of diagnostic accuracy was performed in these two SWE indices. With the use of ROC curves (Figure 5), the optimal cut-off of $E_{maximum}$ and E_{mean} in distinguishing benign and malignant nodules were 67.3 kPa and 23.1 kPa, respectively. Using the optimal cut-off of $E_{maximum}$, 19 malignant and 59 benign nodules were correctly evaluated. The sensitivity, specificity, and overall accuracy of $E_{maximum}$ were 70.4%, 70.2%, and 70.3%, respectively. Using the optimal cut-off of E_{mean}, 20 malignant and 56 benign nodules were correctly assessed, and the sensitivity, specificity, and overall accuracy of E_{mean} were 74.1%, 66.7%, and 68.5%, respectively (Table 2).

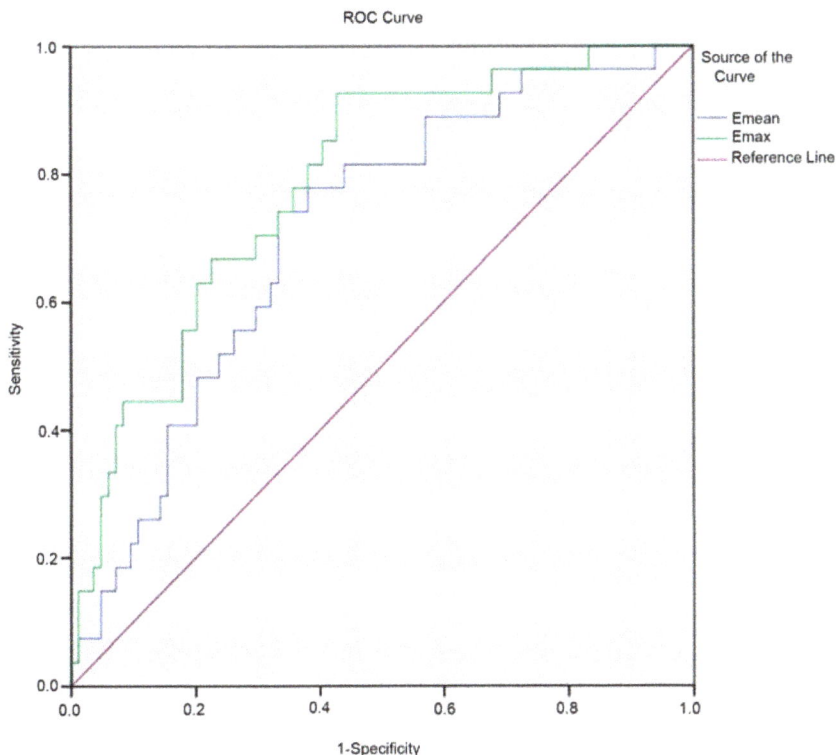

Figure 5. Receiver operating characteristic (ROC) curves used to determine the optimal cut-off level of $E_{maximum}$ and E_{mean} in distinguishing benign and malignant thyroid nodules. Area under the curve, AUC, of E_{mean} and $E_{maximum}$ were 0.71 and 0.785, respectively.

3.4. Combination of Grey Scale Ultrasound and Shear Wave Elastography

Result showed that GSU had a high sensitivity (96.3%) but a low specificity (46.4%), leading to an overall accuracy of 58.5% in assessing thyroid nodules. When GSU combined with SWE ($E_{maximum}$ or E_{mean}), the overall accuracy increased to 80.2% for $E_{maximum}$ and 78.4% for E_{mean} with a sensitivity of 70.4% and 74.1% and specificity of 83.3% and 79.8%, respectively (Table 2, Figure 6). When GSU combined with $E_{maximum}$ or E_{mean}, 19 or 20 malignant and 70 or 67 benign thyroid nodules were correctly identified, respectively.

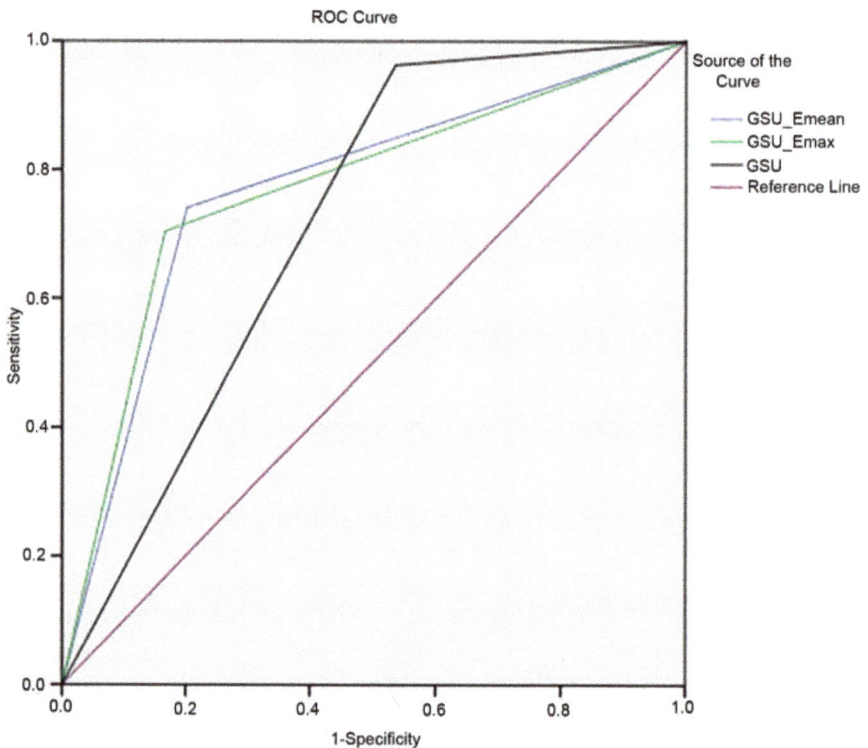

Figure 6. Receiver operating characteristic (ROC) curves showing comparison between grey scale ultrasound features alone (usg. combine) and in combination with $E_{maximum}$ (usg. E_{max}) and E_{mean} (usg. E_{mean}) in distinguishing benign and malignant thyroid nodules. Area under the curve, AUC, of usg. combine, usg. E_{mean}, and usg. $E_{maximum}$ were 0.714, 0.775 and 0.769 respectively.

4. Discussion

Differential diagnosis of thyroid nodules to predict malignancy poses a diagnostic dilemma in clinical settings. FNAC and histopathology examination of surgical specimen of thyroid nodules are the standard procedures to diagnose thyroid cancer. FNAC has a false-positive rate of 1–11.5% and a false-negative rate about 7.7%, whilst 20–30% of cases are non-diagnostic [31,32]. However, the technique is highly dependent on the experience of the pathologists and the adequacy of the samples attained. Moreover, histopathological features of malignant thyroid nodules overlap with benign nodules, and thus there is a high incidence of "skip diagnosis". GSU is commonly used to assess thyroid nodules but no single GSU feature can accurately predict thyroid malignancy [33]. SWE is a novel ultrasound technique that measures tissue elasticity by tracking shear wave propagation through body tissues and provides quantitative measurements. The technique is less operator-dependent and highly reproducible [10]. SWE evaluation of thyroid nodules has been documented. However, the reported cut-off levels to differentiate benign and malignant nodules were variable, which was probably due to different methodologies used in the studies. Among the available literature, the highest cut-off values of SWE indices for evaluating thyroid malignancy were $\geq$95 kPa for $E_{maximum}$, $\geq$85.2 kPa for E_{mean} and $\geq$54.2 kPa for $E_{minimum}$ [34]. However, Bhatia et al. [35] found that E_{mean} of 34.5 kPa or higher was a significant predictor of malignancy with a sensitivity of 52.9% and specificity of 77.8%. Other studies suggested that SWE was useful in differentiating benign and malignant thyroid nodules when the cut-off level of 66 kPa and 65 kPa for $E_{maximum}$ were used, respectively [15,36]. However,

Szczepanek-Parulska et al. [37] found that the threshold value of 50 kPa for $E_{maximum}$ was the most useful SWE parameter in the differentiation of benign and malignant nodules. Using the cut-off value of $\geq$53.2 kPa for $E_{maximum} \geq 34.5$ kPa for E_{mean} and $\geq$21.8 kPa for $E_{minimum}$, Duan et al. [33], found that SWE was superior to conventional GSU in identifying malignant nodules. Among different SWE indices, they found that E_{mean} yielded the highest diagnostic accuracy (79.6%). Liu et al. [13] also reported that $E_{mean} \geq 38.3$ kPa was the most useful predictor among all SWE indices in differentiating benign and malignant thyroid nodule. In the present study, the optimal cut-off for $E_{maximum}$ and E_{mean} for distinguishing benign and malignant nodules were 67.3 and 23.1 kPa, respectively, which were consistent with the result of previous reports in $E_{maximum}$ [15,36]. In our study, there was no significant difference in the $E_{minimum}$ of benign and malignant nodules, which was different from previous studies [13,33,34]. The difference was due to the different methodologies used in the present and previous studies. Previous studies used ROI (Q-box^{TM}) with fixed size and placed it over the stiffer region of the nodule for the stiffness measurement. It involved subjective judgement of the operator in the placement of the ROI. However, the present study adjusted the size of the ROI so that it covered the entire nodule. The process did not involve operator's judgement in which the ROI should be placed, and thus it was more objective. In addition, the method used in the present study allowed for a more comprehensive assessment of the nodule because the ROI covered the entire nodule in the image. Our result suggested that the tissue stiffness within malignant thyroid nodules are varied, with some areas are significantly stiffer than benign nodules (as demonstrated by significantly higher $E_{maximum}$ and E_{mean} in malignant nodules), whereas some areas have similar stiffness as benign nodules (as demonstrated by the similar $E_{minimum}$ between benign and malignant nodules). This may be related to the uneven distribution of tumor cells within the nodule. Results of our study demonstrated that $E_{maximum}$ and E_{mean} are potential predictors for thyroid malignancy when using cut-off value of 67.3 kPa and 23.1 kPa, respectively. However, $E_{minimum}$ has limited value in distinguishing benign and malignant nodules.

In the present study, we evaluated the diagnostic performance of GSU alone and a combination of GSU and SWE. Results showed that the overall diagnostic accuracy of GSU alone was 58.5% and it was increased to 80.2% and 78.4% when it combined with $E_{maximum}$ (cut-off: 67.3 kPa) and E_{mean} (cut-off: 23.1 kPa), respectively. Our results also demonstrated that when GSU combined with SWE, and the specificity increased from 46.4% to 83.3% when using $E_{maximum}$ and to 79.8% when using E_{mean}. However, the sensitivity decreased from 96.3% to 70.4% and 74.1%, respectively. The finding was different from previous reports. In Dobruch-Sobczak et al. [38], they reported that the combination of GSU with SWE did not significantly improve the diagnostic accuracy of malignant thyroid nodules. In the other studies, there was no significant difference in the diagnostic accuracy of GSU alone and combination of GSU and SWE indices in distinguishing benign and malignant thyroid nodules, 86.3% and 87.2% [34]; 81% and 77.9% [39]; and, 60.3% and 60.3% [36], respectively. They also found that when combined GSU with SWE indices the specificity decreased but the sensitivity increased [34,36,39]. One previous study that analysed thyroid nodules in population of France and found that there was an increase in sensitivity from 77.1% to 97.1% however specificity was reduced from 58.0 to 55.3% when grey scale ultrasound was added to $E_{maximum}$ 65 kPa [36]. Similar results were obtained by another investigation conducted on thyroid nodules in Korean population and found that sensitivity was improved from 92.9% to 95% while specificity was reduced from 60.8% to 56.7% on addition of $E_{minimum}$ 85.2 kPa. with grey scale ultrasound [34]. Another study conducted in China found an increase in sensitivity from 76.2% to 87.1%, while specificity was reduced from 83.0 to 73.9 kPa on addition of grey scale ultrasound to $E_{minimum}$ 39.3 kPa [39]. The different result of previous reports and the present study was due to the different criteria in determining malignant thyroid nodules when combined with GSU with SWE. In previous studies, thyroid nodules were malignant when they either had one or more malignant grey scale sonographic features or had a SWE index value greater than the cut-off. This criterion increased the sensitivity by having more true-positive findings, but it also increased the number of false-positive findings leading to decreased specificity [34,36,38,39]. Since the extent of changes of specificity and sensitivity were similar, there was no significant improvement in the overall diagnostic accuracy when GSU combined with SWE in previous reports. However, in the present study, we considered thyroid nodules to be malignant when they had both malignant grey scale sonographic features (one or more features) and had a SWE index value greater than the cut-off. Using this assessment criterion, there was a substantial improvement in specificity with a moderate decrease in sensitivity leading to a significant improvement in the overall accuracy. Using the samples of the present study, the overall diagnostic accuracy was improved from 58.5% to 80.2% in $E_{maximum}$ and to 78.3% in E_{mean}. Although the diagnostic accuracy of combining GSU and SWE in our study was similar to those in previous studies, our study demonstrated substantial improvement in in the diagnostic accuracy after combining the two techniques, whereas previous studies showed no significance difference or decreased in the diagnostic accuracy [34,36,39,40] (Table 4). The similar accuracy of the present study (78.3–80.2%) and previous studies (60.3–87.2%) was probably due to the use of different samples of the patients in the studies. However, we believe that the method that we proposed in our study can enhance the diagnostic accuracy in differential diagnosis of thyroid nodules.

Table 4. Differences in diagnostic accuracy between the results of the present and previous studies to highlight the significant improvement achieved in the current study.

Studies Involved and SWE Index Used	Diagnostic Accuracy (%)		Difference in Diagnostic Accuracy (%)
	GSU Alone	GSU + SWE	
Present study			
$E_{maximum}$ (67.3 kPa)	58.5	80.2	21.7
E_{mean} (23.1 kPa)	58.5	78.3	19.8
Veyrieres et al. [36]			
$E_{maximum}$ (65 kPa)	81	77.9	−3.1
Park et al. [34]			
$E_{minimum}$ (85.2 kPa)	86.3	87.2	0.9
Liu et al. [39]			
$E_{minimum}$ (39.3 kPa)	60.3	60.3	0

In routine clinical thyroid ultrasound examination, operators should consider examining the internal cervical chain to identify any metastatic cervical lymph nodes when malignant thyroid nodule is found. Ultrasound is a useful imaging tool to assess cervical lymph nodes. Metastatic cervical lymph nodes from papillary thyroid carcinoma are usually hyperechoic when compared to adjacent muscles, round in shape, without echogenic hilus, and have punctate calcification [41]. In addition, the combination of ultrasound and computed tomography can help to predict extrathyroidal extension [42], and fluorodeoxyglucose positron emission tomography/computed tomography (FDG-PET/CT) scans should be considered for detecting metastases in post-operative patients with aggressive histology of differentiated thyroid cancer [43].

In the present study, there were 84 benign and 27 malignant thyroid nodules. The calculated power of this sample size in evaluating the performance of GSU and SWE indices in distinguishing benign and malignant thyroid nodules ranged between 0.874 and 0.999 (G*Power version 3.1.9.2, Düsseldorf, Germany). There were limitations in the present study. The majority of the malignant thyroid nodules were papillary thyroid cancer, and thus we did not evaluate the difference of SWE indices among different types of malignant thyroid nodules. Future studies with larger sample size of various types of thyroid cancer can be conducted to investigate the value of SWE in differential diagnosis of different types of thyroid cancer. We did not evaluate the intra-operator and inter-operator reliability in SWE measurement of thyroid nodule stiffness. However, a previous study reported that SWE has satisfactory intra-operator (0.65–0.78) and inter-operator (0.72–0.77) reliability in the evaluation of neck lesions [35].

5. Conclusions

SWE indices (E_{maximum} and E_{mean}) were independent predictors for thyroid malignancy. Combining GSU with SWE indices (using a cutoff of $\geq$67.3 kPa and $\geq$23.1 kPa for E_{maximum} and E_{mean} respectively) can improve the overall diagnostic accuracy in distinguishing benign and malignant thyroid nodules. SWE is a useful adjunct to GSU in the assessment of thyroid nodules.

Acknowledgments: This study was supported by a research grant from The Hong Kong Polytechnic University, Hong Kong (RU55).

Author Contributions: All authors (listed below) have made substantial contribution in this study. M.Y. provided the concept and design of the study. He performed the thyroid ultrasound examinations, and edited the manuscript. F.N.B. performed image and data analyses and wrote the manuscript. S.Y.W.L. helped in recruiting the patients and edited the manuscript. H.-C.L. contributed in performing the inter-observer study. H.K.W.L. and S.-P.Y. revised the manuscript for intellectual content.

Conflicts of Interest: The authors declare no conflict of interest. The founding sponsors had no role in the design of the study; in the collection, analyses, or interpretation of data; in the writing of the manuscript, and in the decision to publish the results.

References

1. Kim, S.-Y.; Kim, E.-K.; Moon, H.J.; Yoon, J.H.; Kwak, J.Y. Application of texture analysis in the differential diagnosis of benign and malignant thyroid nodules: Comparison with gray-scale ultrasound and elastography. *Am. J. Roentgenol.* **2015**, *205*, W343–W351. [CrossRef] [PubMed]

2. Kwak, J.Y.; Kim, E.-K. Ultrasound elastography for thyroid nodules: Recent advances. *Ultrasonography* **2014**, *33*, 75–82. [CrossRef] [PubMed]

3. Chan, B.K.; Desser, T.S.; McDougall, I.R.; Weigel, R.J.; Jeffrey, R.B. Common and uncommon sonographic features of papillary thyroid carcinoma. *J. Ultrasound Med.* **2003**, *22*, 1083–1090. [CrossRef] [PubMed]

4. Cooper, D.S.; Doherty, G.M.; Haugen, B.R.; Kloos, R.T.; Lee, S.L.; Mandel, S.J.; Mazzaferri, E.L.; McIver, B.; Pacini, F.; Schlumberger, M. Revised american thyroid association management guidelines for patients with thyroid nodules and differentiated thyroid cancer: The american thyroid association (ata) guidelines taskforce on thyroid nodules and differentiated thyroid cancer. *Thyroid* **2009**, *19*, 1167–1214. [CrossRef] [PubMed]

5. Moon, W.-J.; Baek, J.H.; Jung, S.L.; Kim, D.W.; Kim, E.K.; Kim, J.Y.; Kwak, J.Y.; Lee, J.H.; Lee, J.H.; Lee, Y.H. Ultrasonography and the ultrasound-based management of thyroid nodules: Consensus statement and recommendations. *Korean J. Radiol.* **2011**, *12*, 1–14. [CrossRef] [PubMed]

6. Cappelli, C.; Castellano, M.; Pirola, I.; Cumetti, D.; Agosti, B.; Gandossi, E.; Rosei, E.A. The predictive value of ultrasound findings in the management of thyroid nodules. *QJM* **2007**, *100*, 29–35. [CrossRef] [PubMed]

7. Frates, M.C.; Benson, C.B.; Charboneau, J.W.; Cibas, E.S.; Clark, O.H.; Coleman, B.G.; Cronan, J.J.; Doubilet, P.M.; Evans, D.B.; Goellner, J.R. Management of thyroid nodules detected at us: Society of radiologists in ultrasound consensus conference statement 1. *Radiology* **2005**, *237*, 794–800. [CrossRef] [PubMed]

8. Cappelli, C.; Castellano, M.; Pirola, I.; Gandossi, E.; De Martino, E.; Cumetti, D.; Agosti, B.; Rosei, E.A. Thyroid nodule shape suggests malignancy. *Eur. J. Endocrinol.* **2006**, *155*, 27–31. [CrossRef] [PubMed]

9. Razavi, S.A.; Hadduck, T.A.; Sadigh, G.; Dwamena, B.A. Comparative effectiveness of elastographic and b-mode ultrasound criteria for diagnostic discrimination of thyroid nodules: A meta-analysis. *Am. J. Roentgenol.* **2013**, *200*, 1317–1326. [CrossRef] [PubMed]

10. Sun, J.; Cai, J.; Wang, X. Real-time ultrasound elastography for differentiation of benign and malignant thyroid nodules. *J. Ultrasound Med.* **2014**, *33*, 495–502. [CrossRef] [PubMed]

11. Haugen, B.R. 2015 american thyroid association management guidelines for adult patients with thyroid nodules and differentiated thyroid cancer: What is new and what has changed? *Thyroid* **2016**, *26*, 1–133. [CrossRef] [PubMed]

12. Hong, Y.; Liu, X.; Li, Z.; Zhang, X.; Chen, M.; Luo, Z. Realeallines for adult patients with thyroid nodules and differentiated thyroidalignant thyroid nodules. *J. Ultrasound Med.* **2009**, *28*, 861–867. [CrossRef] [PubMed]

13. Liu, B.-X.; Xie, X.-Y.; Liang, J.-Y.; Zheng, Y.-L.; Huang, G.-L.; Zhou, L.-Y.; Wang, Z.; Xu, M.; Lu, M.-D. Shear wave elastography versus real-time elastography on evaluation thyroid nodules: A preliminary study. *Eur. J. Radiol.* **2014**, *83*, 1135–1143. [CrossRef] [PubMed]
14. Khoo, M.L.; Asa, S.L.; Witterick, I.J.; Freeman, J.L. Thyroid calcification and its association with thyroid carcinoma. *Head Neck* **2002**, *24*, 651–655. [CrossRef] [PubMed]
15. Sebag, F.; Vaillant-Lombard, J.; Berbis, J.; Griset, V.; Henry, J.; Petit, P.; Oliver, C. Shear wave elastography: A new ultrasound imaging mode for the differential diagnosis of benign and malignant thyroid nodules. *J. Clin. Endocrinol. Metab.* **2010**, *95*, 5281–5288. [CrossRef] [PubMed]
16. Cantisani, V.; Grazhdani, H.; Drakonaki, E.; D'Andrea, V.; Di Segni, M.; Kaleshi, E.; Calliada, F.; Catalano, C.; Redler, A.; Brunese, L. Strain us elastography for the characterization of thyroid nodules: Advantages and limitation. *Int. J. Endocrinol.* **2015**, *2015*, 908575. [CrossRef] [PubMed]
17. Rosario, P.W.; Silva, A.L.D.; Borges, M.A.R.; Calsolari, M.R. Is doppler ultrasound of additional value to gray-scale ultrasound in differentiating malignant and benign thyroid nodules? *Arch. Endocrinol. Metab.* **2015**, *59*, 79–83. [CrossRef] [PubMed]
18. Anil, G.; Hegde, A.; Chong, F. Thyroid nodules: Risk stratification for malignancy with ultrasound and guided biopsy. *Cancer Imaging* **2011**, *11*, 209–223. [PubMed]
19. Khadra, H.; Bakeer, M.; Hauch, A.; Hu, T.; Kandil, E. Is vascular flow a predictor of malignant thyroid nodules? *A meta-analysis. Gland Surg.* **2016**, *5*, 576–582. [CrossRef] [PubMed]
20. Moon, H.J.; Kwak, J.Y.; Kim, M.J.; Son, E.J.; Kim, E.-K. Can vascularity at power doppler us help predict thyroid malignancy? *Radiology* **2010**, *255*, 260–269. [CrossRef] [PubMed]
21. Dudea, S.M.; Botar-Jid, C. Ultrasound elastography in thyroid disease. *Med. Ultrason.* **2015**, *17*, 74. [CrossRef] [PubMed]
22. Kim, E.-K.; Park, C.S.; Chung, W.Y.; Oh, K.K.; Kim, D.I.; Lee, J.T.; Yoo, H.S. New sonographic criteria for recommending fine-needle aspiration biopsy of nonpalpable solid nodules of the thyroid. *Am. J. Roentgenol.* **2002**, *178*, 687–691. [CrossRef] [PubMed]
23. Papini, E.; Guglielmi, R.; Bianchini, A.; Crescenzi, A.; Taccogna, S.; Nardi, F.; Panunzi, C.; Rinaldi, R.; Toscano, V.; Pacella, C.M. Risk of malignancy in nonpalpable thyroid nodules: Predictive value of ultrasound and color-doppler features. *J. Clin. Endocrinol. Metab.* **2002**, *87*, 1941–1946. [CrossRef] [PubMed]
24. Benson, J.; Fan, L. *Tissue Strain Analytics—A Complete Ultrasound Solution for Elastography*; Siemens Healthcare White Paper; Global Siemens Headquaters: Munchen, Germany, 2012.
25. Shiina, T. Jsum ultrasound elastography practice guidelines: Basics and terminology. *J. Med. Ultrason.* **2013**, *40*, 309–323. [CrossRef] [PubMed]
26. Couade, M.; Pernot, M.; Prada, C.; Messas, E.; Emmerich, J.; Bruneval, P.; Criton, A.; Fink, M.; Tanter, M. Quantitative assessment of arterial wall biomechanical properties using shear wave imaging. *Ultrasound Med. Biol.* **2010**, *36*, 1662–1676. [CrossRef] [PubMed]
27. Dighe, M.K. Elastography of thyroid masses. *Ultrasound Clin.* **2014**, *9*, 13–24. [CrossRef] [PubMed]
28. Koperek, O.; Scheuba, C.; Puri, C.; Birner, P.; Haslinger, C.; Rettig, W.; Niederle, B.; Kaserer, K.; Chesa, P.G. Molecular characterization of the desmoplastic tumor stroma in medullary thyroid carcinoma. *Int. J. Oncol.* **2007**, *31*, 59–68. [CrossRef] [PubMed]
29. Popli, M.B.; Rastogi, A.; Bhalla, P.; Solanki, Y. Utility of gray-scale ultrasound to differentiate benign from malignant thyroid nodules. *Indian J. Radiol. Imaging* **2012**, *22*, 63. [CrossRef] [PubMed]
30. Wong, K.; Ahuja, A.T. Ultrasound of thyroid cancer. *Cancer Imaging* **2005**, *5*, 157. [CrossRef] [PubMed]
31. Yoon, J.H.; Kwak, J.Y.; Moon, H.J.; Kim, M.J.; Kim, E.-K. The diagnostic accuracy of ultrasound-guided fine-needle aspiration biopsy and the sonographic differences between benign and malignant thyroid nodules 3 cm or larger. *Thyroid* **2011**, *21*, 993–1000. [CrossRef] [PubMed]
32. Eilers, S.G.; LaPolice, P.; Mukunyadzi, P.; Kapur, U.; Wendel Spiczka, A.; Shah, A.; Saleh, H.; Adeniran, A.; Nunez, A.; Balachandran, I. Thyroid fineinedifferences between benign and malignant thyroid nodules 3 cm or larger. *Cancer Cytopathol.* **2014**, *122*, 745–750. [CrossRef] [PubMed]
33. Duan, S.-B.; Yu, J.; Li, X.; Han, Z.-Y.; Zhai, H.-Y.; Liang, P. Diagnostic value of two-dimensional shear wave elastography in papillary thyroid microcarcinoma. *Onco Targets Ther.* **2016**, *9*, 1311. [PubMed]
34. Park, A.Y.; Son, E.J.; Han, K.; Youk, J.H.; Kim, J.-A.; Park, C.S. Shear wave elastography of thyroid nodules for the prediction of malignancy in a large scale study. *Eur. J. Radiol.* **2015**, *84*, 407–412. [CrossRef] [PubMed]

35. Bhatia, K.S.; Tong, C.S.; Cho, C.C.; Yuen, E.H.; Lee, Y.Y.; Ahuja, A.T. Shear wave elastography of thyroid nodules in routine clinical practice: Preliminary observations and utility for detecting malignancy. *Eur. Radiol.* **2012**, *22*, 2397–2406. [CrossRef] [PubMed]

36. Veyrieres, J.-B.; Albarel, F.; Lombard, J.V.; Berbis, J.; Sebag, F.; Oliver, C.; Petit, P. A threshold value in shear wave elastography to rule out malignant thyroid nodules: A reality? *Eur. J. Radiol.* **2012**, *81*, 3965–3972. [CrossRef] [PubMed]

37. Szczepanek-Parulska, E.; Woliński, K.; Stangierski, A.; Gurgul, E.; Biczysko, M.; Majewski, P.; Rewaj-Łosyk, M.; Ruchała, M. Comparison of diagnostic value of conventional ultrasonography and shear wave elastography in the prediction of thyroid lesions malignancy. *PLoS ONE* **2013**, *8*, e81532. [CrossRef] [PubMed]

38. Dobruch-Sobczak, K.; Zalewska, E.B.; Gumińska, A.; Słapa, R.Z.; Mlosek, K.; Wareluk, P.; Jakubowski, W.; Dedecjus, M. Diagnostic performance of shear wave elastography parameters alone and in combination with conventional b-mode ultrasound parameters for the characterization of thyroid nodules: A prospective, dual-center study. *Ultrasound Med. Biol.* **2016**, *42*, 2803–2811. [CrossRef] [PubMed]

39. Liu, B.; Liang, J.; Zheng, Y.; Xie, X.; Huang, G.; Zhou, L.; Wang, W.; Lu, M. Two-dimensional shear wave elastography as promising diagnostic tool for predicting malignant thyroid nodules: A prospective single-centre experience. *Eur. Radiol.* **2015**, *25*, 624–634. [CrossRef] [PubMed]

40. Dong, M.-J.; Liu, Z.-F.; Zhao, K.; Ruan, L.-X.; Wang, G.-L.; Yang, S.-Y.; Sun, F.; Luo, X.-G. Value of 18f-fdg-pet/pet-ct in differentiated thyroid carcinoma with radioiodine-negative whole-body scan: A meta-analysis. *Nucl. Med. Commun.* **2009**, *30*, 639–650. [CrossRef] [PubMed]

41. Ahuja, A.; Chow, L.; Chick, W.; King, W.; Metreweli, C. Metastatic cervical nodes in papillary carcinoma of the thyroid: Ultrasound and histological correlation. *Clin. Radiol.* **1995**, *50*, 229–231. [CrossRef]

42. Lee, D.Y.; Kwon, T.-K.; Sung, M.-W.; Kim, K.H.; Hah, J.H. Prediction of extrathyroidal extension using ultrasonography and computed tomography. *Int. J. Endocrinol.* **2014**, *2014*, 351058. [CrossRef] [PubMed]

43. Nascimento, C.; Borget, I.; Al Ghuzlan, A.; Deandreis, D.; Hartl, D.; Lumbroso, J.; Berdelou, A.; Lepoutre-Lussey, C.; Mirghani, H.; Baudin, E. Postoperative fluorine-18-fluorodeoxyglucose positron emission tomography/computed tomography: An important imaging modality in patients with aggressive histology of differentiated thyroid cancer. *Thyroid* **2015**, *25*, 437–444. [CrossRef] [PubMed]

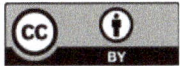

© 2017 by the authors. Licensee MDPI, Basel, Switzerland. This article is an open access article distributed under the terms and conditions of the Creative Commons Attribution (CC BY) license (http://creativecommons.org/licenses/by/4.0/).

applied
sciences

MDPI

Article

Interpretation US Elastography in Chronic Hepatitis B with or without Anti-HBV Therapy

Cheng-Han Lee [1], Yung-Liang Wan [2,3], Tse-Hwa Hsu [1], Shiu-Feng Huang [4], Ming-Chin Yu [5], Wei-Chen Lee [6], Po-Hsiang Tsui [3], Yi-Cheng Chen [1], Chun-Yen Lin [1] and Dar-In Tai [1,*]

[1] Department of Gastroenterology and Hepatology, Chang Gung Memorial Hospital, Taipei 105, Taiwan; b9102011@cgmh.org.tw (C.-H.L.); echohsuth45@cgmh.org.tw (T.-H.H.); yicheng@cgmh.org.tw (Y.-C.C.); chunyenlin@gmail.com (C.-Y.L.)

[2] Department of Medical imaging and Intervention, Chang Gung Memorial Hospital, Taoyuan 333, Taiwan; ylw0518@cgmh.org.tw

[3] Department of Medical imaging and Radiological Sciences, College of Medicine, Institute for Radiological Research, Chang Gung University, Taoyuan 333, Taiwan; tsuiph@mail.cgu.edu.tw

[4] Division of Molecular and Genomic Medicine, National Health Research Institute, Taipei 115, Taiwan; sfhuang@nhri.org.tw

[5] Department of General Surgery, Chang Gung Memorial Hospital, Taoyuan 333, Taiwan; a75159@cgmh.org.tw

[6] Department of Liver and Transplantation Surgery, Chang Gung Memorial Hospital, Taoyuan 333, Taiwan; weichen@cgmh.org.tw

* Correspondence: tai48978@cgmh.org.tw; Tel.: +886-3328-1200 (ext. 8107)

Received: 15 September 2017; Accepted: 30 October 2017; Published: 13 November 2017

Abstract: Inflammation has significant impacts on liver fibrosis measurement by ultrasound elastography. The interpretation requires further optimization in patients with or without anti-viral therapy. We prospectively enrolled a consecutive series of patients with chronic hepatitis B who received liver histology analysis and acoustic radiation force impulse (ARFI). 146 patients who underwent liver biopsy (50.9%) or tumor resection (49.1%) were enrolled. 34 patients (23.3%) had been receiving anti-hepatitis B therapy of various duration. The areas under the receiver-operating characteristic (AUROC) for the diagnosis of Metavir F4 by mean ARFI was 0.820 in the non-treatment group and 0.796 in the treatment group. The ARFI tended to be not lower (100%) than the corresponding Metavir grading in patients with treatment within 12 months, equal (75%) from 13 to 31 months, and lower (71.4%) after 32 months. We conclude that ARFI is a reliable tool for measurement of liver fibrosis in chronic hepatitis B patients with ALT (alanine aminotransferase) <5x the upper limit of normal. For those patients under anti-HBV therapy, the optimal timing for ARFI analysis will be over 1–2.5 years of nucleos(t)ide analogue therapy. The ARFI measurement after 2.5 years tends to be lower than the corresponding histology grading.

Keywords: acoustic radiation force impulse; chronic hepatitis B; liver cirrhosis; anti-HBV therapy

1. Introduction

Liver cirrhosis is the major risk factor for mortality in chronic hepatitis B carriers [1,2]. The annual rate of progression from chronic hepatitis to cirrhosis is 2–5% in hepatitis B e antigen-positive and 3–10% in e antigen-negative patients [3,4]. Patients with absent or low-grade fibrosis at diagnosis are thought to have a relatively lower risk of progression to cirrhosis in 20 years [5]. The diagnosis and further therapeutic decision usually relies on the fibrosis severity, so an accurate assessment is crucial to treatment outcomes. It is easy to diagnose cirrhosis by liver ultrasound [1,2]—what is more difficult is assessing more subtle degrees of fibrosis. Liver biopsy is considered the gold standard for liver fibrosis assessment; however, it is an invasive procedure with rare, but serious complications (mortality rate < 0.01%) [6]. Sampling error and intra- or inter-observer variability also affect the diagnostic consistency [7]. Elastography, either by transient elastography or acoustic radiation force impulse (ARFI), is a promising, non-invasive modality for the diagnosis of liver fibrosis [8–11]. It can be performed in a periodic follow-up and is generally superior to other serological modalities [12–14]. In a meta-analysis study, ARFI demonstrated a satisfactory ability to predict higher-stage liver fibrosis (F = 3) and liver cirrhosis (F = 4) [15]. However, inflammation, variation, and other factors have significant impacts on the interpretation [16–22]. In our previous study as well as in others, ARFI had a poorer performance in the measurement of liver fibrosis in chronic hepatitis B than in chronic hepatitis C [16]. How to make interpretation of liver fibrosis during anti-HBV therapy is unclear. To improve the interpretation of ARFI in chronic hepatitis B patients with or without anti-HBV therapy, we conducted a replication study using two-location measurements and limited the operator to one well-trained technician.

2. Materials and Methods

2.1. Study Design and Subjects

A consecutive series of patients with liver diseases who received liver biopsy or segmental hepatectomy at Chang Gung Memorial Hospital, Linkou Medical Centre from January 2014 to December 2016 were enrolled prospectively.

We included all patients who were seropositive for hepatitis B surface antigen and age greater than 18-year-old in this study. The following patients were excluded: (i) those co-infected with hepatitis C virus or human immunodeficiency virus (HIV) infection, or presenting autoimmune or alcoholic liver disease; (ii) those with liver cirrhosis, functional classification Child B or C; (iii) those with a liver tumor greater than 5 cm in the R hepatic lobe, which makes ARFI unable to select a suitable location for measurement, and (iv) those who refused to sign an inform consent form.

All of the patients from the outpatient department received ARFI on the day of the liver biopsy. For those hospitalized patients planning to receive surgery for tumor resection, ARFI was performed within one month before the surgery.

This study was approved by the Institute Review Board of Chang Gung Memorial Hospital (IRB: 104-2353C). Written Informed consent was obtained from all participants before the start of the study.

2.2. Laboratory Assessments

Blood samples were obtained under fasting conditions. Liver biochemistry, the international normalized ratio (INR) of prothrombin time (PT), and a hemogram were measured using commercially available kits and automatic analyzers. HBsAg and anti-HCV were tested with an enzyme immunoassay (Abbott Diagnostics). The entire study was conducted in the clinical laboratory of this hospital, a laboratory certified by The College of American Pathologists.

2.3. Serology Tests for Fibrosis

The aspartate to platelet ratio index (APRI) [23] and the fibrosis-4 score (FIB4) [24] are used as non-invasive serology methods to measure liver fibrosis. The APRI was calculated using the formula: (Aspartate Aminotransferase (AST) [U/L]/upper limit of normal [U/L]) $\times$ (100/platelet [109/L]).

The FIB-4 values were calculated using the formula: age (years) $\times$ AST [U/L]/(platelets [109/L] $\times$ Alanine Aminotransferase (ALT) [U/L])1/2).

2.4. Histological Assessment

Each patient from the outpatient department was initially screened by hemogram, prothrombin time, and blood biochemistry to ensure that there was no contraindication for liver biopsies. US-guided percutaneous liver biopsy was performed using an 18-gauge biopsy core needle with an automatic pistol device (Bard Magnum, Bard Peripheral Vascular Inc., Tempe, AZ, USA). For patients who had received surgical resection, the resected non-tumor part was used for liver fibrosis assessment. The tissue samples were fixed with formalin and embedded with paraffin, and 4-μm-thick sections were stained with hematoxylin and eosin (H&E) and reticulin silver (Masson trichome method). Histology was evaluated by an experienced pathologist (S.-F.H.) who was unaware of the ARFI study. Liver fibrosis stages were evaluated semi-quantitatively according to the Metavir scoring system [25]. Necroinflammatory activity was graded according to the modified histological activity index grading system (Ishak) in 4 categories: A for periportal or periseptal interface hepatitis; B for confluent necrosis; C for focal lytic necrosis, apoptosis, and focal inflammation; and D for portal inflammation with a maximal score of 18 [26].

2.5. ARFI Imaging Study

ARFI imaging was mainly carried out with Acuson S2000 (Siemens Healthcare, Erlangen, Germany) and Virtual Touch tissue quantification software (Siemens Healthcare). The study protocol was generally according to the guideline with some modification [27]. Most of the examinations were conducted by one experienced technician (H.-T.W.). On a few occasions, the study was conducted by experienced hepatologists (D.-I.T. or Y.-C.C.). They were unaware of the patients' histology during ARFI measurements. The patients remained supine with the right arm extended above the head during the scan. All of the patients received ARFI measurements from the right intercostal space. We selected two locations separated by one intercostal space featuring optimal real-time ultrasonography with liver tissue having no large blood vessels [16]. Location A targeted the right lower liver, while Location B targeted the right upper liver. During the measuring process, the area of interest was maintained at a vertical angle to the skin. A measurement with a depth of 3–6 cm beneath the skin was chosen to standardize the examination. Most patients were asked to maintain a normal, slow breath during the measurement. In patients with rapid breathing, temporary holding of the breath during the measurement was requested. Valsalva Maneuver, which causes reduction of hepatic venous blood flow may decrease liver stiffness. No patients encountered failure of assessment for shortness of breathing. At least 10 measurements were obtained for each location. Liver stiffness measurements were considered valid only if 10 successful acquisitions were obtained, and the interquartile range (IQR) to median ratio of the 10 acquisitions was <0.25. When data from two locations had a difference greater than 0.2 m/sec, repeat measurements were taken to confirm the study [28].

2.6. FibroScan

A FibroScan 502 touch machine (Echosens®, Paris, France) has been available in our hospital since July 2016. Both ARFI and transient elastography were done at the same time to all patients enrolled in the last 6 months of the study. M probe was used for measurement in all of the patients. For those patients with a body mass index greater than 28, an extra large (XL) probe was performed. All procedures were performed by a well-trained technician according to the relevant manufacturers.

2.7. Statistics

Patient characteristics were expressed as the number and percentage or mean ± standard deviation (SD) as appropriate. Continuous variables of two independent groups were compared with a Student's t-test or Mann–Whitney U test depending on the distribution. Categorical variables were tested using the chi-square test or Fisher's exact test, as applicable. The receiver-operating characteristic (ROC) curves and areas under the ROC (AUROC) were calculated for evaluation of the best prediction tests for histology proven liver cirrhosis. All statistical analyses were performed using SPSS (version 11.5; SPSS Inc., Chicago, IL, USA) or Interactive Chi-square Test to calculate the difference between groups (Preacher, KJ. Calculation for the chi-square test: An interactive calculation tool for chi-square tests of goodness of fit and independence, http://quantpsy.org). A *p* value of <0.05 was considered to indicate statistical significance.

The case numbers needed for AUROC analysis to reach type I error 0.05 and type II error (1-power) 0.20 was calculated by MedCalc-version 16.8 (MedCalc Software bvba, Oostende, Belgium). When the AUROC curve is expected to be 0.8 and null hypothesis value is 0.5, the minimal case numbers needed to achieve statistic power 0.8 will be around 27 cases.

3. Results

3.1. Patient Demographics

A total of 146 patients with chronic hepatitis B were enrolled. The demographic characteristics are shown in Table 1. Seventy-four (50.9%) patients underwent liver needle biopsy and seventy-two patients (49.1%) received liver tumor resection. Thirty-four patients (23.3%) had been receiving anti-HBV therapy of varying duration at the time of enrollment. The mean age of all patients was 53.0 ± 10.7 years. The male gender was predominant in both groups (82.4% in treatment group vs. 75.9% in non-treatment). The treatment group had a lower platelet count (161.62×10^9/L vs. 187.33×10^9/L, $p = 0.034$), a lower Ishak's inflammation score (2.76 vs. 3.89, $p = 0.020$), and a higher ultrasound fibrosis score (7.26 vs. 6.43, $p = 0.001$) than the non-treatment group Twenty-four patients (21.4%) in the non-treatment group and 14 patients (41.2%) in the treatment group had histologically proven liver cirrhosis (Metavir fibrosis score = 4).

Table 1. Demographic and laboratory data with or without anti-HBV therapy.

Category	Non-Treatment	Treatment	p Value #
Total No	112	34	
Age (year)	52.34 ± 10.80	55.05 ± 10.41	
Male (%)	85 (75.9)	28 (82.4)	
Liver cancer (%)	55 (49.1)	19 (55.9)	
Ultrasound spleen index (cm^2)	16.58 ± 7.10	16.84 ± 5.80	
Ultrasound fibrosis score	6.43 ± 1.38	7.26 ± 1.05	0.001
GGT (glutamyl transpetidase) (U/L)	60.9 ± 71.68	56.48 ± 53.90	
AST (U/L)	73 ± 111	49 ± 48	
ALT (U/L)	92 ± 193	56 ± 75	
Bilirubin (mg/DL)	0.97 ± 1.22	0.76 ± 0.36	
Platelet (10^9/L)	187.33 ± 65.10	161.62 ± 47.52	0.034
Prothrombin time (* INR)	1.07 ± 0.08	1.08 ± 0.06	
Body height (cm)	164.56 ± 7.51	164.81 ± 10.47	
Body weight (kg)	69.38 ± 10.47	69.45 ± 13.30	
Histology			
Ishak inflammatory score	3.89 ± 2.45	2.76 ± 1.74	0.020
Confluence necrosis (No.)	3 (2.7)	1 (2.9)	
Metavir fibrosis score 0	3 (2.7)	0 (0)	
Metavir fibrosis score 1	12 (10.7)	2 (5.9)	
Metavir fibrosis score 2	43 (38.4)	5 (14.7)	
Metavir fibrosis score 3	30 (26.8)	13 (38.2)	
Metavir fibrosis score 4	24 (21.4)	14 (41.2)	0.026

Number in the parenthesis is percentage of total cases. * INR = international normalized ratio; # Univariate analysis, not significant after multivariate analysis.

3.2. Sensitivity and Specificity of ARFI Measurements

Data on ARFI were successfully obtained by two-location measurements from all patients. The diagnostic performance of ARFI and serum fibrosis markers for liver fibrosis was assessed using ROC curves. According to the data on two-location measurements, ARFI values measured at Location A or B, mean values of Locations A and B, and higher or lower ARFI data between Locations A and B were examined separately.

For comparison with ARFI parameters, data on APRI and FIB4 were combined in the ROC curve analysis. The results are listed in Figure 1 for patients without anti-HBV therapy and in Figure 2 for patients with anti-HBV therapy. The ARFI-related parameters have significantly higher area under the ROC (AUROC) curve than APRI or FIB4 in both treatment and non-treatment groups.

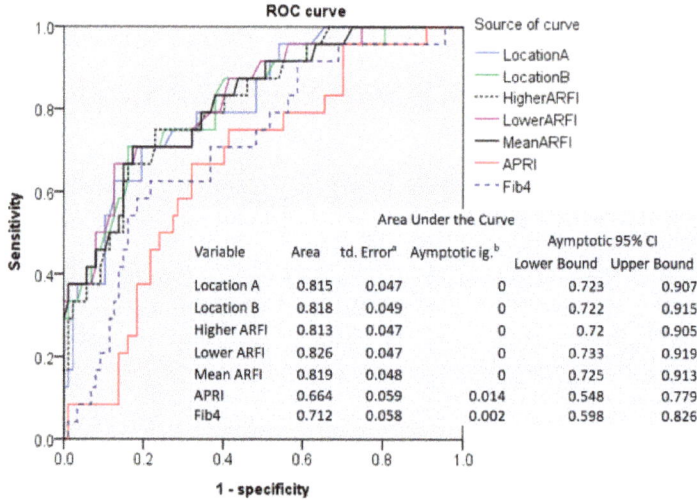

Source of curve: LocationA, LocationB, HigherARFI, LowerARFI, MeanARFI, APRI, Fib4

Area Under the Curve

Variable	Area	td. Error[a]	Aymptotic ig.[b]	Aymptotic 95% CI Lower Bound	Upper Bound
Location A	0.815	0.047	0	0.723	0.907
Location B	0.818	0.049	0	0.722	0.915
Higher ARFI	0.813	0.047	0	0.72	0.905
Lower ARFI	0.826	0.047	0	0.733	0.919
Mean ARFI	0.819	0.048	0	0.725	0.913
APRI	0.664	0.059	0.014	0.548	0.779
Fib4	0.712	0.058	0.002	0.598	0.826

Figure 1. The areas under the receiver-operating characteristic (AUROC) of acoustic radiation force impulse (ARFI) values, APRI, and fibrosis-4 score (FIB4) for prediction of liver cirrhosis in patients with chronic hepatitis B without anti-HBV therapy. A higher AUROC is found in ARFI-related parameters (0.813~0.826) than in APRI (0.664) or FIB4 (0.712) (Aymptotic 95% CI: Asymptotic 95% Confidence Intervals; [a] Standard Error; [b] Asymptotic *p* value).

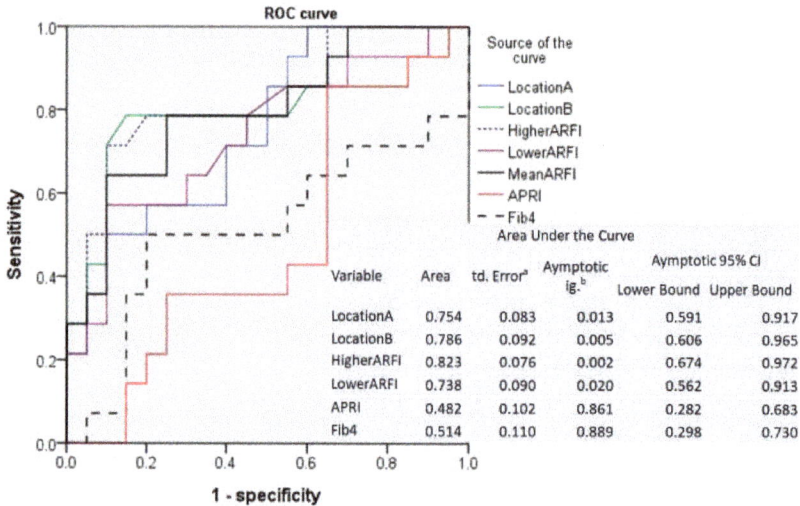

Source of the curve: LocationA, LocationB, HigherARFI, LowerARFI, MeanARFI, APRI, Fib4

Area Under the Curve

Variable	Area	td. Error[a]	Aymptotic ig.[b]	Aymptotic 95% CI Lower Bound	Upper Bound
LocationA	0.754	0.083	0.013	0.591	0.917
LocationB	0.786	0.092	0.005	0.606	0.965
HigherARFI	0.823	0.076	0.002	0.674	0.972
LowerARFI	0.738	0.090	0.020	0.562	0.913
APRI	0.482	0.102	0.861	0.282	0.683
Fib4	0.514	0.110	0.889	0.298	0.730

Figure 2. The AUROC of ARFI values, APRI, and FIB4 for prediction of liver cirrhosis in patients with chronic hepatitis B with anti-HBV therapy. A higher AUROC is found in ARFI-related parameters (0.737~0.823) than in APRI (0.482) or FIB4 (0.514) (Aymptotic 95% CI: Asymptotic 95% Confidence Intervals; [a] Standard Error; [b] Asymptotic *p* value).

According to the results of AUROC analysis, the cut-off values for the prediction of liver cirrhosis on each parameter are listed in Table 2. Among the ARFI parameters, lower ARFI shows the highest AUROC curve (0.827) in non-treatment groups, whereas higher ARFI shows the highest AUROC curve (0.823) in the treatment group. To simplify the cut-off system, we use mean ARFI in both treatment and non-treatment groups.

The AUROC for the diagnosis of Metavir F4 by mean ARFI is 0.820 [standard error of mean (SE) 0.048, (confidence intervals (CI): 0.725; 0.913) Figure 1] in the non-treatment group. The cut-off value for the prediction of liver cirrhosis (Metavir F4) by mean ARFI is 1.523 m/sec with a sensitivity of 0.708 and a specificity of 0.830 in the non-treatment group (Table 2). Since inflammation has a significant impact on ARFI value, AUROC was performed on 99 patients with an ALT level lower than 5x upper limit normal (ULN). The cut-off values remain almost the same (1.523) with increasing sensitivity (0.696) and specificity (0.829). When only the 79 patients with an ALT level lower than 2x ULN were included, the AUROC showed a similar cut-off value (1.523) without a significant improvement in sensitivity and specificity as compared with those patients with an ALT lower than 5x ULN.

The AUROC for the diagnosis of Metavir F4 by mean ARFI is 0.796 [SE 0.080, (CI: 0.641; 0.952) Figure 2] in the treatment group. The cut-off value of mean ARFI for diagnosis of liver cirrhosis was 1.420 m/sec with a sensitivity of 0.786 and a specificity of 0.750 in the treatment group (Table 2).

Table 2. Cut-off values in different ARFI measurements for Metavir 4 in patients with difference inflammation.

Type of ARFI	AUROC	Cut-Off (m/sec)	Sensitivity	1-Specificity
Patients without anti-HBV treatment (N = 112)				
Location A	0.816	1.505	0.708	0.193
Location B	0.818	1.515	0.708	0.159
Higher	0.813	1.515	0.750	0.227
Lower	0.827	1.460	0.708	0.182
Mean	0.820	1.523	0.708	0.170
Patients without anti-HBV treatment and ALT level <5x ULN (N = 99)				
Location A	0.816	1.415	0.739	0.263
Location B	0.815	1.460	0.739	0.263
Higher	0.793	1.485	0.739	0.257
Lower	0.827	1.460	0.696	0.184
Mean	0.818	1.523	0.696	0.171
Patients without anti-HBV treatment and ALT level <2x ULN (N = 79)				
Location A	0.789	1.415	0.706	0.258
Location B	0.761	1.460	0.647	0.274
Higher	0.764	1.520	0.647	0.258
Lower	0.793	1.460	0.647	0.177
Mean	0.775	1.523	0.647	0.177
Patients with anti-HBV treatment (N = 34)				
Location A	0.754	1.495	0.571	0.200
Location B	0.786	1.480	0.786	0.150
Higher	0.823	1.515	0.768	0.200
Lower	0.737	1.490	0.571	0.100
Mean	0.796	1.420	0.786	0.250

3.3. Correlation of Histological Metavir Scores with Mean ARFI Value

The mean ARFI value increased with the progression of the histological Metavir scoring system in both treatment and non-treatment groups. A significant correlation was found between the two variables in the non-treatment group (Spearman's rho correlation coefficients 0.597, $p < 0.001$) and in the treatment group (Spearman's rho correlation coefficients 0.587, $p < 0.001$, Figure 3).

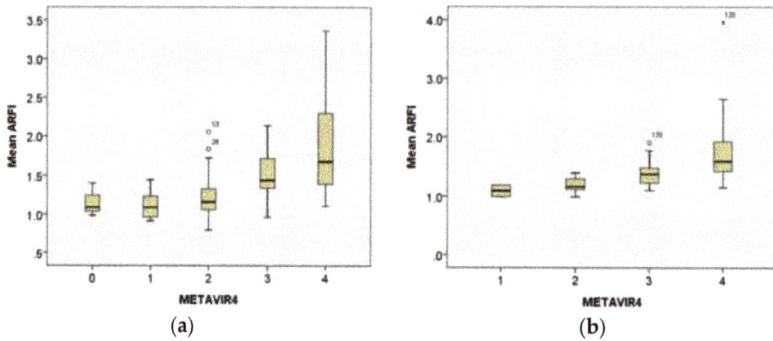

(a)   (b)

Figure 3. Mean ARFI values of each METAVIR fibrosis score. A significant correlation was found between mean ARFI values with Metavir grading in the non-treatment group ((**a**) Sperman's rho correlation coefficients 0.597, $p < 0.001$) and treatment group ((**b**) Sperman's rho correlation coefficients 0.587, $p < 0.001$).

3.4. Correlation of ARFI with FibroScan

Twenty-seven patients had undergone both ARFI and FibroScan studies. All of these patients did not receive anti-HBV therapy at the time of elastography study. The correlation of mean ARFI with FibroScan is quite high. The Pearson correlation is 0.794 with a p-value < 0.001 (Figure 4).

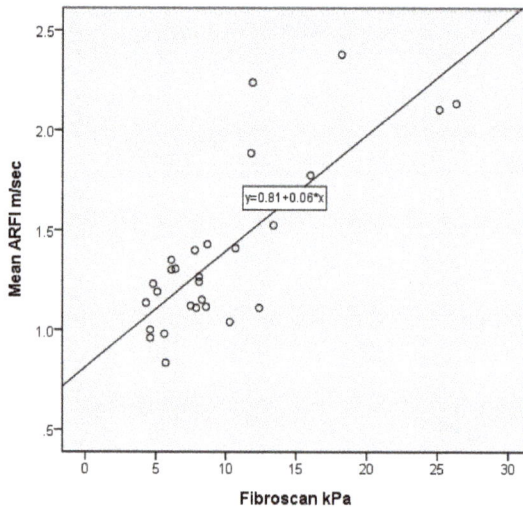

Figure 4. Correlation of Mean ARFI with FibroScan in 27 cases without anti-HBV therapy. The Pearson correlation is 0.794 with a $p < 0.001$ (2-tailed).

3.5. Correlation of ARFI Values with Metavir Score and Treatment Duration

In the treatment group (Table 3), 19 of the 34 patients (55.9%) received segmentectomy for hepatocellular carcinoma (HCC). All of them had been receiving anti-HBV therapy at the time of histology analysis and ARFI study. Twenty-two patients (64.7%) received Entecavir, eight (23.5%) received Tenofovir, two (5.9%) received Telbivudine, one (2.9%) received pegylated interferon 2a, and one (2.9%) received Adefovir/Telbivudine combination therapy.

The mean ARFI was negatively correlated with treatment duration (Spearman's rho correlation coefficients -0.428, $p < 0.012$). According to our unpublished experiences for those patients with chronic hepatitis B with an ALT level lower than 180 IU/L, the cut-off values for prediction of Metavir fibrosis scores 0, 1, 2, 3, 4 are 1.105, 1.218, 1.343, and 1.478 m/sec, respectively. When ARFI predicted that Metavir fibrosis scores were correlated with histology Metavoir score and duration of therapy, the ARFI value tended to be equal (3/5, 60%) or higher (2/5, 40%) than the corresponding Metavir score for treatment duration within 12 months, equal between 13 and 31 months (9/12, 75%), and frequently lower (12/17, 71.4%) for treatment duration greater or equal to 32 months ($p = 0.0012$, Table 3).

Table 3. Correlation of ARFI, Metavir score, and treatment duration.

Case	Age	Sex	HCC	ALT	Durg	Treatment (Mo)	METAVIR	# Mean of Two Locations	* Predicted Metavir Score	** Compared with Histology Metavir Score
T1	55.7	M	1	48	ETV	2	2	1.17	2	equal
T2	48.3	M	0	335	Pegasy	5	2	1.4	3	higher
T3	52.8	M	0	103	ETV	6	2	1.3	2	equal
T4	47.3	M	0	50	ETV	12	3	1.5	4	higher
T5	30.2	M	0	46	ETV	12	4	1.84	4	equal
T6	50.3	M	0	100	TDF	13	3	1.41	3	equal
T7	45.2	M	0	39	ETV	14	4	1.59	4	equal
T8	71.3	F	0	172	ETV	18	4	3.96	4	equal
T9	52.1	M	0	23	ETV	19	3	1.77	4	higher
T10	64.1	F	1	23	ETV	21	3	1.38	3	equal
T11	55.3	M	1	45	ETV	22	4	1.73	4	equal
T12	53.0	M	1	19	ADVTBV	26	4	1.59	4	equal
T13	57.1	M	1	42	ETV	28	3	1.15	1	lower
T14	60.9	M	1	16	ETV	29	4	1.93	4	equal
T15	65.6	F	0	10	ETV	31	3	1.49	4	higher
T16	64.0	F	1	27	TDF	31	4	2.65	4	equal
T17	45.9	M	0	26	ETV	31	4	2.12	4	equal
T18	51.5	M	1	26	ETV	32	3	1.29	3	lower
T19	41.3	M	1	26	ETV	32	4	1.43	2	lower
T20	49.3	M	0	35	TDF	36	3	1.47	1	lower
T21	68.4	F	1	19	TDF	36	4	1.16	2	lower
T22	45.4	M	1	45	TDF	36	3	1.29	3	equal
T23	45.0	M	0	316	TDF	37	4	1.9	4	equal
T24	68.1	M	0	16	ETV	39	1	0.995	0	lower
T25	59.7	M	0	34	TDF	39	3	1.36	3	equal
T26	42.0	M	0	19	ETV	41	3	1.105	1	lower
T27	60.3	M	1	50	TDF	44	2	1.12	1	lower
T28	63.0	F	1	16	TBV	48	2	0.995	0	lower
T29	73.9	M	1	13	TBV	52	4	1.52	4	equal
T30	62.7	M	1	26	ETV	55	3	1.23	2	lower
T31	38.5	M	1	26	ETV	58	4	1.18	1	lower
T32	50.4	M	1	24	ETV	60	1	1.19	1	equal
T33	63.7	M	1	21	ETV	68	3	1.115	1	lower
T34	69.5	M	1	68	ETV	71	4	1.435	3	lower

T8: possible hypoglycemic agent related toxic hepatitis; T23: poor compliance. Abbreviation: ADV (adefovir); ETV (entecavir); TBV (telbivudine); TDF (tenofovir); # Spearman's rho correlation coefficients -0.428, $p < 0.012$. * The cut-off values for prediction of Metavir fibrosis scores 0, 1, 2, 3, 4 are 1.105, 1.218, 1.343, 1.478 m/sec, respectively. ** Chi-square test of goodness of fit and independence $p = 0.0012$.

4. Conclusions

We collected a series of 146 patients with chronic hepatitis B who underwent liver needle biopsy (50.9%) or surgery for tumor resection (49.1% Table 1). Thirty-four (23.3%) patients had received anti-HBV therapy at the time of liver histology and ARFI analysis. The AUROC for mean ARFI (0.796, Figure 2) to detect liver cirrhosis (Metavir F4) in anti-HBV treated patients. When the cut-off of the mean ARFI was set to 1.420 m/sec, the sensitivity was 0.786 and the specificity was 0.750 (Table 2). To the best of our knowledge, the correlation between histology and ARFI in patients receiving anti-HBV treatment was quite rare and was generally in HIV/HBV dual-infected patients [29,30].

The main reason for this lower ARFI cut-off level was the suppression of liver inflammation by anti-HBV therapy [31,32]. ARFIs and FibroScans measure liver stiffness by shear-wave velocity. Both of them are greatly influenced by inflammation [33,34]. This is especially a problem in patients with chronic hepatitis B [16]. The inflammatory activity in chronic hepatitis B is not constant and is characterized by intermittent acute exacerbation [35]. There is additional problem in this study: we included patients with hepatocellular carcinoma. ARFI may miss a tumor area according to imaging that is more suitable than the FibroScan in the present study.

We correlated ARFI with Metavir score over different durations of treatment. The values of ARFI tended to be higher than those of histology when the duration of treatment was shorter than or equal to 12 months (Table 3). This could have been because inflammation was not completely suppressed. The ARFI was correlated rather well with the Metavir score between 12 and 31 months after treatment. At this period, the inflammation was suppressed to a minimal level, as evidenced by a low ALT level in most cases. Therefore, the optimal timing for ARFI to measure liver fibrosis will be the second year of nucleos(t)ide analogues therapy. After that, the ARFI level tended to be lower than the histological fibrosis grading. These biases were not related to the small liver sample. Most of the mismatches between ARFI and histology were patients of HCC. These findings indicated that a decrease in liver stiffness identified by ARFI precedes the morphological changes of fibrosis. These observations also confirm that the improvement in liver stiffness at the initial stage is mainly due to reduced necroinflammation [36].

In the non-treatment group, the AUROC of lower ARFI was 0.827 (Figure 1), which was better than that in our previous study (lower ARFI AUROC: 0.707) [16]. Both studies used two-location measurements. This difference may be related to a lower level of inflammation in the current study than in the previous study. The previous study enrolled patients with chronic hepatitis B who intended to receive anti-HBV therapy. In this study, most of the patients were HCC who were hospitalized for surgical resection. The ALT level was lower in this study than in the previous study (91.90 IU/L vs. 117.19 IU/L). The other major difference was that a single operator performed most of the measurements in this study, while the previous study was conducted by several hepatologists. We believe that it is essential to measure ARFI using a standardized protocol and to limit the operator to one or two well-trained, full-time technicians. These measures may decrease the variation and make the data more reliable. In 27 patients in this series, both Fibrosan and ARFI two-location measurements are employed. The correlation is quite good (Figure 4; Pearson correlation: 0.794).

For those patients without anti-HBV therapy, a simple way to reduce the influence of inflammation is to exclude patients with a high ALT level. After excluding those with an ALT level greater than 5x ULN, we found that the cut-off value for diagnosis of liver cirrhosis was similar to that of the entire series (Table 2). However, the sensitivity and specificity are improved. Further reduction or ALT level to 2x ULN did not improve the sensitivity or the specificity. It is our limitation that ALT is a somewhat indirect marker of liver inflammation. Other serological markers of liver inflammation could potentially help to select patients for ARFI studies.

We excluded patients with advance cirrhosis. Our cut-off value was lower than most of the studies in Western countries [9,10,22]. However, the cut-off value is similar to reports from Korea [37] and China with low ALT levels [38]. Therefore, we set the mean ARFI cut-off value for liver cirrhosis to be 1.523 m/sec for the non-treatment group. For patients receiving anti-HBV therapy, the cut-off value will be lower than untreated patients and is treatment duration dependence.

The other limitation of our study is that we did not have enough cases to present longitudinal results. We only collected ARFI data before and during various durations of anti-viral treatment in our patients. We will evaluate the long-term result after a suitable number of cases have been collected.

We conclude that ARFI is a reliable tool for the measurement of liver fibrosis in chronic hepatitis B with low inflammation status. For those patients with active inflammation, the optimal timing for ARFI analysis will be within the second year of nucleos(t)ide analogue therapy.

Acknowledgments: This study was funded in full by Chang Gung Memorial Hospital, grant number CMRPG3F0331 and CMRPG3E1121.

Author Contributions: Study concept and design: D.-I.T.; acquisition of data: T.-H.H.; participation in patient management and data collection: T.-H.H., M.-C.Y., W.-C.L., P.-H.T., Y.-C.C., and C.-Y.L.; histology reading: S.-F.H.; statistical analysis, interpretation of data, and drafting of the manuscript: D.-I.T. and C.-H.L.; critical review of the manuscript: Y.-L.W. All authors reviewed the paper and approved the final version.

Conflicts of Interest: The authors have no financial or personal relationships with other people or organizations that could have inappropriately influenced their work.

Abbreviations

ARFI   acoustic radiation force impulse
ALT   alanine aminotransferase
HCV   hepatitis C virus
HBV   hepatitis B virus
HIV   human immunodeficiency virus
INR   international normalized ratio
PT   prothrombin time
FIB4   Fibrosis-4 Score
ROC   receiver-operating characteristic
AUROC   areas under ROC

References

1. Tai, D.I.; Lin, S.M.; Sheen, I.S.; Chu, C.M.; Lin, D.Y.; Liaw, Y.F. Long-term outcome of hepatitis B e antigen-negative hepatitis B surface antigen carriers in relation to changes of alanine aminotransferase levels over time. *Hepatology* **2009**, *49*, 1859–1867. [CrossRef] [PubMed]

2. Tai, D.I.; Tsay, P.K.; Chen, W.T.; Chu, C.M.; Liaw, Y.F. Relative Roles of HBsAg seroclearance and mortality in the decline of HBsAg prevalence with increasing age. *Am. J. Gastroenterol.* **2010**, *105*, 1102–1109. [CrossRef] [PubMed]

3. Fattovich, G.; Bortolotti, F.; Donato, F. Natural history of chronic hepatitis B: Special emphasis on disease progression and prognostic factors. *J. Hepatol.* **2008**, *48*, 335–352. [CrossRef] [PubMed]

4. Liaw, Y.F. Natural history of chronic hepatitis B virus infection and long-term outcome under treatment. *Liver Int.* **2009**, *29*, 100–107. [CrossRef] [PubMed]

5. Sebastiani, G.; Gkouvatsos, K.; Pantopoulos, K. Chronic hepatitis C and liver fibrosis. *World J. Gastroenterol.* **2014**, *20*, 11033–11053. [CrossRef] [PubMed]

6. Bravo, A.A.; Sheth, S.G.; Chopra, S. Liver biopsy. *N. Engl. J. Med.* **2001**, *344*, 495–500. [CrossRef] [PubMed]

7. Regev, A.; Berho, M.; Jeffers, L.J.; Milikowski, C.; Molina, E.G.; Pyrsopoulos, N.T.; Feng, Z.Z.; Reddy, K.R.; Schiff, E.R. Sampling error and intraobserver variation in liver biopsy in patients with chronic HCV infection. *Am. J. Gastroenterol.* **2002**, *97*, 2614–2618. [CrossRef] [PubMed]

8. Friedrich-Rust, M.; Ong, M.F.; Martens, S.; Sarrazin, C.; Bojunga, J.; Zeuzem, S.; Herrmann, E. Performance of transient elastography for the staging of liver fibrosis: A meta-analysis. *Gastroenterology* **2008**, *134*, 960–974. [CrossRef] [PubMed]

9. Bota, S.; Herkner, H.; Sporea, I.; Salzl, P.; Sirli, R.; Neghinal, A.M.; Peck-Radosavljevic, M. Meta-analysis: ARFI elastography versus transient elastography for the evaluation of liver fibrosis. *Liver Int.* **2013**, *33*, 1138–1147. [CrossRef] [PubMed]

10. Kircheis, G.; Sagir, A.; Vogt, C.; Vom Dahl, S.; Kubitz, R.; Häussinger, D. Evaluation of acoustic radiation force impulse imaging for determination of liver stiffness using transient elastography as a reference. *World J. Gastroenterol.* **2012**, *18*, 1077–1084. [CrossRef] [PubMed]

11. Lee, S.; Kim, D.Y. Non-invasive diagnosis of hepatitis B virus-related cirrhosis. *World J. Gastroenterol.* **2014**, *20*, 445–459. [CrossRef] [PubMed]

12. Crespo, G.; Fernández-Varo, G.; Mariño, Z.; Casals, G.; Miquel, R.; Martinez, S.M.; Gilabert, R.; Forns, X.; Jimenez, W.; Navasa, M. ARFI, FibroScan, ELF, and their combinations in the assessment of liver fibrosis: A prospective study. *J. Hepatol.* **2012**, *57*, 281–287. [CrossRef] [PubMed]

13. Tapper, E.B.; Afdhal, N.H. Vibration-controlled transient elastography: A practical approach to the noninvasive assessment of liver fibrosis. *Curr. Opin. Gastroenterol.* **2015**, *31*, 192–198. [CrossRef] [PubMed]

14. Ferraioli, G.; Filice, C.; Castera, L.; Choi, B.I.; Sporea, I.; Wilson, S.R.; Cosgrove, D.; Dietrich, C.F.; Amy, D.; Bamber, J.C.; et al. WFUMB guidelines and recommendations for clinical use of ultrasound elastography Part 3: Liver. *Ultrasound Med. Biol.* **2015**, *41*, 1161–1179. [CrossRef] [PubMed]

15. Hu, X.D.; Qiu, L.Y.; Liu, D.; Qian, L.X. Acoustic radiation force impulse elastography for non-invasive evaluation of hepatic fibrosis in chronic hepatitis B and C patients: A systematic review and meta-analysis. *Med. Ultrason.* **2017**, *19*, 23–31. [CrossRef] [PubMed]

16. Tai, D.I.; Tsay, P.K.; Jeng, W.J.; Weng, C.C.; Huang, S.F.; Huang, C.H.; Lin, S.M.; Chiu, C.T.; Chen, W.T.; Wan, Y.L. Differences in liver fibrosis between patients with chronic hepatitis B and C: Evaluation by acoustic radiation force impulse measurements at 2 locations. *J. Ultrasound Med.* **2015**, *34*, 813–821. [CrossRef] [PubMed]

17. Chen, S.H.; Li, Y.F.; Lai, H.C.; Kao, J.T.; Peng, C.Y.; Chuang, P.H.; Su, W.P.; Chiang, I.P. Effects of patient factors on noninvasive liver stiffness measurement using acoustic radiation force impulse elastography in patients with chronic hepatitis C. *BMC Gastroenterol.* **2012**, *12*, 105. [CrossRef] [PubMed]

18. Bota, S.; Sporea, I.; Sirli, R.; Popescu, A.; Danila, M.; Costachescu, D. Intra- and interoperator reproducibility of acoustic radiation force impulse (ARFI) elastography—preliminary results. *Ultrasound Med. Biol.* **2012**, *38*, 1103–1108. [CrossRef] [PubMed]

19. Piscaglia, F.; Salvatore, V.; Di Donato, R.; D'Onofrio, M.; Gualandi, S.; Gallotti, A.; Sagrini, E. Accuracy of VirtualTouch Acoustic Radiation Force Impulse (ARFI) imaging for theet al diagnosis of cirrhosis during liver ultrasonography. *Ultraschall Med. Eur. J. Ultrasound* **2011**, *32*, 167–175. [CrossRef] [PubMed]

20. Liu, K.; Bui, K.T.; Corte, C.; Lee, A.; Ngu, M.C.; Pattullo, V. Longer duration of transient elastography predicts unreliable liver stiffness measurements. *Eur. J. Gastroenterol. Hepatol.* **2015**, *27*, 655–659. [CrossRef] [PubMed]

21. Wong, V.W.; Lampertico, P.; de Lédinghen, V.; Chang, P.E.; Kim, S.U.; Chen, Y.P.; Chan, H.L.Y.; Mangia, G.; Foucher, J.; Chow, W.C.; et al. Probability-based interpretation of liver stiffness measurement in untreated chronic hepatitis B patients. *Dig. Dis. Sci.* **2015**, *60*, 1448–1456. [CrossRef] [PubMed]

22. Song, P.; Mellema, D.C.; Sheedy, S.P.; Meixner, D.D.; Karshen, R.M.; Urban, M.W.; Manduca, A.; Sanchez, W.; Callstrom, M.R.; Greenleaf, J.F.; et al. Performance of 2-Dimensional Ultrasound Shear Wave Elastography in Liver Fibrosis Detection Using Magnetic Resonance Elastography as the Reference Standard: A Pilot Study. *J. Ultrasound Med.* **2016**, *35*, 401–412. [CrossRef] [PubMed]

23. Wai, C.T.; Greenson, J.K.; Fontana, R.J.; Kalbfleisch, J.D.; Marrero, J.A.; Conjeevaram, H.S.; Lok, A.S.F. A simple noninvasive index can predict both significant fibrosis and cirrhosis in patients with chronic hepatitis C. *Hepatology* **2003**, *38*, 518–526. [CrossRef] [PubMed]

24. Vallet-Pichard, A.; Mallet, V.; Nalpas, B.; Verkarre, V.; Nalpas, A.; Dhalluin-Venier, V.; Fontaine, H.; Pol, S. FIB-4: An inexpensive and accurate marker of fibrosis in HCV infection. Comparison with liver biopsy and fibrotest. *Hepatology* **2007**, *46*, 32–36. [CrossRef] [PubMed]

25. Bedossa, P.; Poynard, T. An algorithm for the grading of activity in chronic hepatitis C: The METAVIR Cooperative Study Group. *Hepatology* **1996**, *24*, 289–393. [CrossRef] [PubMed]

26. Ishak, K.; Baptista, A.; Bianchi, L.; Callea, F.; De Groote, J.; Gudat, F.; Denk, H.; Desmet, V.; Korb, G.; MacSween, R.N.M.; et al. Histological grading and staging of chronic hepatitis. *J. Hepatol.* **1995**, *22*, 696–699. [CrossRef]

27. Dietrich, C.F.; Bamber, J.; Berzigotti, A.; Bota, S.; Cantisani, V.; Castera, L.; Cosgrove, D.; Ferraioli, G.; Friedrich-Rust, M.; Gilja, O.H.; et al. EFSUMB Guidelines and Recommendations on the Clinical Use of Liver Ultrasound Elastography, Update 2017 (Long Version). *Ultraschall Med. Eur. J. Ultrasound* **2017**, *38*, e16–e47. [CrossRef] [PubMed]

28. Tai, D.I. Reply. *Ultrasound Med.* **2016**, *35*, 668. [CrossRef] [PubMed]

29. Miailhes, P.; Pradat, P.; Chevallier, M.; Lacombe, K.; Bailly, F.; Cotte, L.; Trabaud, M.-A.; Boibieux, A.; Bottero, J.; Trepo, C.; et al. Proficiency of transient elastography compared to liver biopsy for the assessment of fibrosis in HIV/HBV-coinfected patients. *J. Viral. Hepat.* **2011**, *18*, 61–69. [CrossRef] [PubMed]

30. Maida, I.; Soriano, V.; Castellares, C.; Ramos, B.; Sotgiu, G.; Martin-Carbonero, L.; Barreiro, P.; Rivas, P.; Fonzalez-Lahoz, J.; Nunez, M. Liver fibrosis in HIV-infected patients with chronic hepatitis B extensively exposed to antiretroviral therapy with anti-HBV activity. *HIV Clin. Trials* **2006**, *7*, 246–250. [CrossRef] [PubMed]

31. Lai, C.L.; Shouval, D.; Lok, A.S.; Chang, T.T.; Cheinquer, H.; Goodman, M.D.; Deheertogh, D.; Wilber, R.; Zink, R.C.; Cross, A.; et al. Entecavir versus lamivudine for patients with HBeAg-negative chronic hepatitis B. *N. Engl. J. Med.* **2006**, *354*, 1011–1020. [CrossRef] [PubMed]

32. Chang, T.T.; Gish, R.G.; de Man, R.; Gadano, A.; Sollano, J.; Chao, Y.C.; Lok, A.S.; Han, K.H.; Goodman, Z.; Zhu, J.; et al. A comparison of entecavir and lamivudine for HBeAg-positive chronic hepatitis B. *N. Engl. J. Med.* **2006**, *354*, 1001–1010. [CrossRef] [PubMed]

33. Viganò, M.; Massironi, S.; Lampertico, P.; Iavarone, M.; Paggi, S.; Pozzi, R.; Conte, D.; Colombo, M. Transient elastography assessment of the liver stiffness dynamics during acute hepatitis B. *Eur. J. Gastroenterol. Hepatol.* **2010**, *22*, 180–184. [CrossRef] [PubMed]

34. Verveer, C.; Zondervan, P.E.; ten Kate, F.J.W.; Hansen, B.E.; Janssen, H.L.A. Evaluation of transient elastography for fibrosis assessment compared with large biopsies in chronic hepatitis B and C. *Liver Int.* **2012**, *32*, 622–628. [CrossRef] [PubMed]

35. Liaw, Y.F.; Tai, D.I.; Chu, C.M.; Pao, C.C.; Chen, T.J. Acute exacerbation in chronic type B hepatitis: Comparison between HBeAg and antibodypositive patients. *Hepatology* **1987**, *7*, 20–23. [CrossRef] [PubMed]

36. Knop, V.; Hoppe, D.; Welzel, T.; Vermehren, J.; Herrmann, E.; Vermehren, A.; Friedrich-Rust, M.; Sarrazin, C.; Zeuzem, S.; Welker, M.-W. Regression of fibrosis and portal hypertension in HCV-associated cirrhosis and sustained virologic response after interferon-free antiviral therapy. *J. Viral. Hepat.* **2016**, *23*, 994–1002. [CrossRef] [PubMed]

37. Chung, J.H.; Ahn, H.S.; Kim, S.G.; Lee, Y.N.; Kim, Y.S.; Jeong, S.W.; Jang, J.Y.; Lee, S.H.; Kim, H.S.; Kim, B.S. The usefulness of transient elastography, acoustic-radiation-force impulse elastography, and real-time elastography for the evaluation of liver fibrosis. *Clin. Mol. Hepatol.* **2013**, *19*, 156–164. [CrossRef] [PubMed]

38. Zhang, D.; Chen, M.; Wang, R.; Liu, Y.; Zhang, D.; Liu, L.; Zhou, G. Comparison of acoustic radiation force impulse imaging and transient elastography for non-invasive assessment of liver fibrosis in patients with chronic hepatitis B. *Ultrasound Med. Biol.* **2015**, *41*, 7–14. [CrossRef] [PubMed]

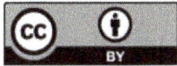

© 2017 by the authors. Licensee MDPI, Basel, Switzerland. This article is an open access article distributed under the terms and conditions of the Creative Commons Attribution (CC BY) license (http://creativecommons.org/licenses/by/4.0/).

applied
sciences

MDPI

Article

Effect of HCV Core Antigen and RNA Clearance during Therapy with Direct Acting Antivirals on Hepatic Stiffness Measured with Shear Wave Elastography in Patients with Chronic Viral Hepatitis C

Mariusz Łucejko and Robert Flisiak *

Department of Infectious Diseases and Hepatology, Medical University of Bialystok, 14 Zurawia St; 15-540 Bialystok, Poland; mariusz.lucejko@gmail.com.
* Correspondence: robert.flisiak@umb.edu.pl; Tel. +48-60-520-3525; Fax: +48-85-741-6921

Received: 19 December 2017; Accepted: 26 January 2018; Published: 29 January 2018

Abstract: To assess a combination of novel measures of therapeutic success in the treatment of chronic hepatitis C (CHC) infection, we evaluated liver stiffness (LS) with shear wave elastography and hepatitis C virus core antigen (HCVcAg) concentrations. We followed 34 patients during and after treatment with direct acting antivirals. All patients achieved a sustained virologic and serologic response and a significant increase of albumin levels. Decreases of alanine aminotransferase (ALT) activity and alpha-fetoprotein (AFP) level were observed during the treatment and follow-up period. A significant decrease in LS was observed between baseline, end of treatment (EOT), and at 24- and 96-week post-treatment follow-up. LS decline between EOT and 96-week follow-up (FU96) was observed in 79% of patients. Significant LS changes were seen in patients with advanced fibrosis, particularly in cirrhotics and in patients with ALT exceeding 100 IU/mL. There was a positive correlation between ALT activity and LS changes at the baseline versus FU96. A negative correlation was demonstrated between individual HCVcAg baseline concentrations and reduction of LS at the baseline versus FU96. In conclusion, we observed that LS significantly declined during and after antiviral treatment. It was accompanied by improvement in some liver function measures, and disappearance of both HCVcAg and HCV ribonucleic acid (HCV RNA).

Keywords: viral hepatitis C; HCV core antigen; shear wave elastography; therapy; direct acting antivirals

1. Introduction

Prevalence of hepatitis C virus (HCV) infection is currently estimated to be 1%, corresponding to about 70 million viremic people worldwide [1]. HCV infection untreated for many years can lead to serious consequences such as liver cirrhosis, hepatocellular carcinoma (HCC), hepatic decompensation and death.

Currently available treatment with direct-acting antivirals (DAAs) is pangenotypic, safe, easy, and short, and its efficacy is almost 100% [2,3].

Diagnosis of HCV infection currently is based on the presence of antibodies followed by HCV RNA detection. According to recent findings, HCV core antigen (HCVcAg) testing can replace HCV RNA detection [4–6]. Its clearance during DAA therapy can predict sustained virologic response (SVR), which is an indicator of HCV clearance [7]. Quantitative HCV RNA is still a gold standard for monitoring anti-viral treatment efficacy. According to the most recent guidelines of the European Association for the Study of the Liver (EASL) the use of HCVcAg was recommended as an alternative marker of treatment efficacy [8]. Since HCVcAg has not been routinely applied for monitoring of treatment efficacy up to now, we decided to use it simultaneously with HCV RNA in our study.

Evaluation of the progression of liver disease is a crucial element of HCV diagnosis, treatment prioritization and its monitoring. Invasiveness, cost and possible side effects of liver biopsy, recognized up to now as a gold standard, have led recently to the rapid development of non-invasive techniques for the evaluation of liver fibrosis [9–12]. Two major directions in this area are serologic tests, combining a number of laboratory measures with a final calculation of the numeric value and measurement of liver stiffness (LS) with transient elastography (TE) or shear wave elastography (SWE) [13,14]. Major advantages of LS measurement are safety, non-invasiveness, the possibility of testing in real time, repeatability and low cost of examination [15–17]. The main weakness of all non-invasive techniques is insufficient differentiation between moderate degrees of fibrosis [18]. However, it is essential to highlight that LS does not represent fibrosis directly; as a matter of fact, the LS value is a resultant of fibrosis, inflammation and blood microcirculation with a possible additional effect of hepatic steatosis or other hepatic conditions, and therefore can serve as an independent measure of liver disease progression [19].

Currently, LS testing is widely used to assess liver disease for possible prioritization of HCV treatment. It can also provide prognostic information during the post-treatment follow-up [20,21]. Some recent studies confirmed higher diagnostic value of SWE compared to TE, and therefore we applied this technique in our practice and in this study [22,23].

Currently, three techniques are available for elastography of the liver: one-dimensional transient elastography, (1D-TE), acoustic radiation force impulse (ARFI) that include point shear wave elastography (pSWE), and real-time two-dimensional shear wave elastography (2D-SWE). Depending on the method used, the shear wave measurement takes place perpendicular to the plane of excitation (pSWE; 2D-SWE) or parallel to excitation (1D-TE). In 1D-TE, the mechanical vibrator exerts a controlled vibrating external "blow" on the surface of the body, which create shear waves which propagate through the examined tissue. After that, the same probe measures the velocity of the shear wave and, after transformation, we get a measurement of stiffness. In pSWE, acoustic radiation force impulse is used to induce tissue movement in the normal direction in a single focal location, but tissue transposition is not measured itself. Longitudinal waves are converted to shear waves through the absorption of acoustic energy; then, the speed of these waves is measured and transformed to quantify tissue elasticity. In the case of 2D SWE, multiple focal zones are examined in rapid series, forming cylindrical shear wave cone and allowing real-time monitoring of shear waves. After transformation, we get color, quantitative elastogram applied to a B-mode image. pSWE and 2D-SWE can be performed using a conventional ultrasound machine in contrast to 1D-TE [24].

Since both HCVcAg and SWE can be considered novel measures of therapeutic success and possible predictors of further outcome of liver disease, we assessed the association between HCVcAg clearance and LS in CHC patients treated with DAAs.

2. Materials and Methods

2.1. Patients

Thirty-four patients with chronic hepatitis C infection were included in the study. All patients were Caucasians: 12 females and 22 males with a median age of 50 (IQR 41.5-58.5). The most common HCV genotype was 1b—demonstrated in 29 (88%) patients, which is consistent with the epidemiological situation in the region of the study [25]. Nineteen (58%) patients had experienced previous interferon-based therapy and 15 (46%) had liver cirrhosis. More details of baseline patients' characteristics are presented in Table 1. HCV infection was confirmed in all patients according to a common diagnostic algorithm (presence of serum anti-HCV antibody and HCV RNA). Patients with HIV (human immunodeficiency virus) or HBV (hepatitis B virus) co-infection, pregnant or planning pregnancy females, patients with decompensated liver disease (Child-Pugh C class) or with contraindications to planned treatment were excluded from the study.

The study protocol was approved by the Ethics Committee and written informed consent was obtained from each patient before the start of the study.

Table 1. Baseline characteristics.

Characteristics	All; N = 34
Age, years [median (IQR)]	50 (41.5–58.5)
Males [n; %]	10; 59
BMI, kg/m^2 [median (IQR)]	26.2 (23.2–28.6)
HCV RNA, log10 IU/mL [median (IQR)]	5.9 (5.6–6.3)
HCVcAg, fmol/L [median (IQR)]	2653 (1168–4716)
HCV genotype 1a/1b/3a/4 [%]	6/88/0/6
Prior HCV treatment history	-
null response [n; %]	8; 24
partial response [n; %]	4; 12
relapse [n; %]	9; 26
naive [n; %]	12; 35
unknown [n; %]	1; 3
PLT—× 10^3 cell/mm^3 [median (IQR)]	154 (91–201)
Hemoglobin—g/dL [median (IQR)]	15.1 (13.73–15.9)
Albumin—mg/dL [median (IQR)]	4.3 (3.9–4.7)
ALT—IU/mL [median (IQR)]	75.5 (40.3–140)
Bilirubin—mg/dL [median (IQR)]	0.7 (0.5–0.9)
AFP—ng/dL [median (IQR)]	6.2 (2.8–20.2)
Liver stiffness—kPa [median (IQR)]	10.2 (7.8–17.9)
Liver cirrhosis [n;%]	14; 42
MELD score [median (min–max)]	7 (6–15)
Child Pugh score [median (min–max)]	5 (5–9)

BMI—body mass index; HCV RNA; ribonucleic acid hepatitis C virus; HCVcAg—hepatitis C core antigen; PLT—platelets; ALT—alanine aminotransferase; AFP—alpha-fetoprotein; kPa-kilopascal; MELD—Model of End-Stage Liver Disease; IQR—interquartile range; log10—decimal logarithm.

2.2. Treatment Regimens

Twenty-four patients were treated with fixed doses of ombitasvir/paritaprevir/ritonavir possibly combined with dasabuvir and ribavirin (OBV/PRV/r ± DSV ± RBV) and ten patients with ledipasvir/sofosbuvir (LDV/SOF) according to product characteristics, EASL and national guidelines [26]. Selection of the medication for a particular patient was based on the physician's judgment.

2.3. Study Design

Blood samples for HCV RNA, HCVcAg and laboratory measures of hepatic function were collected during the treatment and follow-up period at the baseline, end of treatment (EOT), and follow-up 24 weeks (FU24) and 96 weeks (FU96) after treatment termination. Sustained virologic response (SVR) was defined as undetectable serum HCV RNA 24 weeks after treatment termination, and sustained serologic response (SSR) was defined as HCVcAg undetectability.

2.4. HCV RNA and HCVcAg Measurement

Blood samples were collected in EDTA (ethylenediaminetetraacetic acid) containing tubes and plasma was separated. Plasma samples for HCV RNA and HCVcAg measurements were stored at −70 °C until the time of testing. Serum HCV RNA quantitative levels were determined by a Roche COBAS AmpliPrep HCV test (Roche Molecular System, Pleasanton, CA, USA) with level of quantification 15 IU/mL, and level of detection 11 IU/mL. For quantification of serum HCV core antigen (HCVcAg) samples were tested with the fully automated Architect HCVcAg assay (Abbott Diagnostics, Chicago, IL, USA) according to the manufacturer's recommendations. Concentration of HCVcAg was expressed in femtomoles (fmol/L) per liter (1.0 fmol/L = 0.02 pg/mL). According to the manufacturer, the detection cut-off for a negative value was 3.0 fmol/L, the gray zone was 3–10 fmol/L and the upper detection limit was 180,000 fmol/L. HCV genotype was determined by direct sequencing of the PCR (polymerase chain reaction) product using genotype-specific primers.

2.5. Other Laboratory Measures

Several laboratory measures of hepatic function, including activity of alanine aminotransferase (ALT) and alkaline phosphatase (ALP), concentrations of bilirubin, albumins, alpha-fetoprotein (AFP), creatinine, international normalized ratio (INR), as well as hemoglobin level (Hb) and platelet count (PLT), were analyzed at the baseline, during the treatment and at follow-up visits. Child–Pugh and MELD (model of end-stage liver disease) scores were calculated based on clinical and laboratory measures.

2.6. Liver Stiffness

LS was measured with non-invasive, real-time, quantitative shear wave elastography (2D-SWE) using AIXPLORER equipment (Super Sonic Imagine, Aix-en-Provence, France), with a convex broadband probe (SC6-1) [27,28]. Measurement was carried out according to the protocol provided by the manufacturer. During one SWE examination, three to five successive measurements were taken and the mean expressed in kPa (kilopascal) was documented as the final result. LS values were additionally expressed in the METAVIR scale corresponding to histologic fibrosis according to the manufacturer's recommendations, as follows F0/1: <7.1 kPa, F2: 7.1–8.6 kPa, F3: 8.7–10.3 kPa, F4: >10.4 kPa.

2.7. Statistical Analysis

Statistical analysis was performed with Statistica 10 (StatSoft, Cracow, Poland). Patients' data are presented as the number and percentage, median and interquartile range (IQR). Correlations were analyzed with Spearman's rank correlation coefficient. The normality of the distribution was assessed by the D'Agostino–Pearson test and Shapiro–Wilk test. Differences between groups were assessed by Wilcoxon's signed rank test, the unpaired T-test, and in the case of three or more groups by repeated-measures ANOVA. Differences were considered significant at p values below 0.05.

3. Results

The baseline LS measured in all patients was 14.9 ± 13.2 kPa, and varied from 4.1 to 68.0 kPa. It was significantly ($p = 0.003$) higher in treatment experienced (median 12.6 kPa; IQR 10.1–20.7), than in treatment naïve patients (median 7.9 kPa; IQR 6.6–9.2). According to the METAVIR score, 15 patients (44%) were classified as F4, 7 (21%) F3, 7 (21%) F2 and 5 (15%) F0/1. All patients achieved SVR and SSR. As shown in Table 2, a statistically significant increase of albumin levels, and a decrease of ALT activity and AFP level were observed during the treatment and follow-up period. A statistically significant decrease in LS was observed between baseline and all following time points after treatment termination (Table 3). Moreover, significant differences were also noted between EOT and FU96, as well as between FU24 and FU96. As shown in Figure 1, a decrease in LS between EOT and FU96 was observed in 27 (79%) patients. In analysis based on baseline fibrosis stage, statistically significant changes in LS were seen in patients with advanced fibrosis of F3 and F4 only (Figure 2), and the LS decline was significantly bigger in cirrhotics compared to patients with less advanced disease (Figure 3). LS reduction between baseline and FU96 was significantly ($p = 0.047$) bigger in experienced (median 3.5 kPa; IQR 1.2–8.1), compared to treatment naïve patients (median 0.8 kPa; IQR 0.2–3). The decrease in LS was also significantly ($p = 0.0006$) bigger in patients with ALT exceeding 100 IU/mL (9.27 ± 9.01 kPa) than in those with lower ALT activities (1.42 ± 2.06 kPa). There was also a positive correlation between ALT activity and change in LS at baseline versus FU96 ($r = 0.49$; $p = 0.004$) (Figure 4). As shown in Figure 5, a statistically significant negative correlation ($r = -0.3893$; $p = 0.002$) was also demonstrated between individual HCVcAg baseline concentrations and reduction of LS values at baseline versus FU96.

Table 2. Dynamics of changes in laboratory test and liver stiffness during the treatment and follow-up period; p was calculated with Wilcoxon signed rank.

N = 34	Baseline	EOT	p	FU24	p	FU96	p
[me dian; IQR]	-	-	baseline vs. EOT	-	baseline vs. FU24	-	baseline vs. FU96
HCV RNA log10 IU/mL	5.9 (5.6–6.3)	0	<0.0001	0	<0.0001	0	<0.0001
HCVcAg fmol/L	2653 (1168–4716)	0	<0.0001	0	<0.0001	-	-
Albumin mg/dL	4.3 (3.9–4.7)	4.5 (4.2–4.8)	0.05	4.8 (4.4–5)	<0.0001	4.7 (4.5–4.9)	<0.0001
Bilirubin mg/dL	0.7 (0.5–0.9)	0.7 (0.4–1.2)	ns	0.6 (0.4–0.8)	0.008	0.6 (0.4–0.9)	0.05
Creatinine mg/dL	0.685 (0.585–0.765)	0.715 (0.610–0.810)	0.08	0.725 (0.623–0.803)	0.03	0.820 (0.745–0.890)	<0.0001
Liver stiffness kPa	10.2 (7.8–17.9)	9.8 (6.5–13.9)	0.008	9.1 (6.8–15.6)	0.008	8.2 (5.9–13.2)	<0.0001
ALT IU/mL	75.5 (40.25–140)	24 (16–30.25)	<0.0001	22 (15.75–32.25)	<0.0001	-	-
PLT × 10³ cell/mm³	154 (91–201)	167 (108.3–219.5)	0.04	155 (97.8–207.5)	ns	-	-
Hemoglobin g/dL	15.1 (13.7–15.9)	14.1 (12.5–15.6)	0.009	15.1 (14.1–16.4)	ns	-	-
AFP ng/dL	6.2 (2.8–20.2)	3.3 (2.3–4.7)	<0.0001	3.4 (2.4–4.8)	<0.0001	-	-

EOT—end of treatment; FU24—follow-up visit at week 24 after treatment; FU96—follow-up visit at week 96 after treatment; BMI—body mass index; HCV RNA—ribonucleic acid hepatitis C virus; HCVcAg—hepatitis C core antigen; kPa-kilopascal; ALT—alanine aminotransferase; PLT—platelets; AFP—alpha-fetoprotein.

Table 3. Statistical significance of differences calculated with Wilcoxon signed rank test (p), between LS values at particular examination time points.

p-Values	Baseline	EOT	FU24	FU96
baseline	x	x	x	x
EOT	0.008	x	x	x
FU24	0.008	0.09	x	x
FU96	<0.0001	0.0002	0.005	x

EOT—end of treatment; FU24—follow-up visit at week 24 after treatment; FU96—follow-up visit at week 96 after treatment.

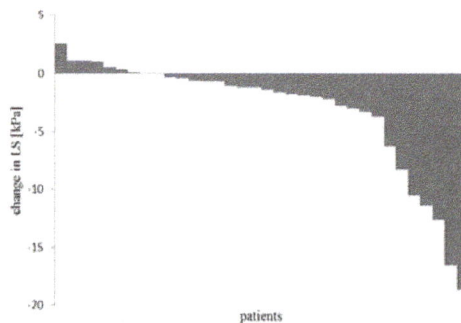

Figure 1. Reduction of liver stiffness between EOT and FU96 in individual patients. Each column represents one patient and the change in liver stiffness between end of treatment and 96 weeks later. LS—liver stiffness; kPa—kilopascal.

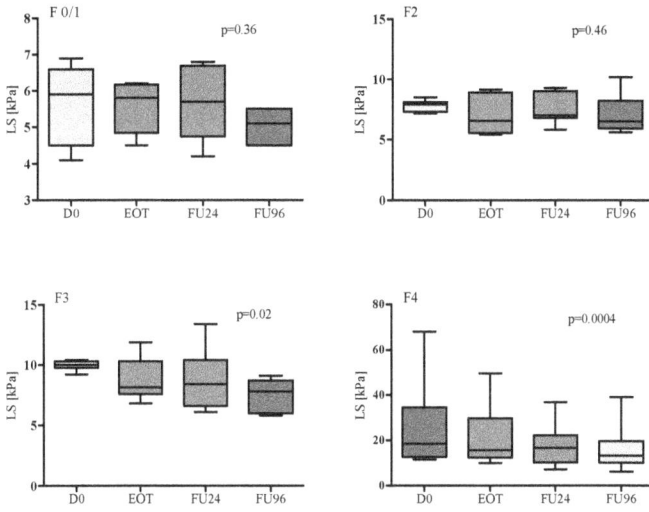

Figure 2. Median values of sequential LS measurement according to baseline fibrosis stage. EOT—end of treatment; FU24—follow-up visit at week 24 after treatment; FU96—follow-up visit at week 96 after treatment; F0/1–F4: METAVIR scores; LS—liver stiffness; kPa—kilopascal; the upper and bottom side of each box represent 25th and 75th percentile (interquartile range); the line passing through the field indicates the median; whiskers indicate minimum and maximum. Statistical method: analysis of variance ANOVA.

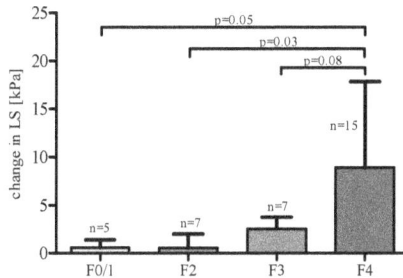

Figure 3. Change in LS after 96 weeks in patients with fibrosis stage F4 and below F4 measured at baseline (unpaired *t*-test). F0/1–F4: METAVIR scores; LS—liver stiffness; kPa—kilopascal; data presented as mean; whiskers indicate standard deviations.

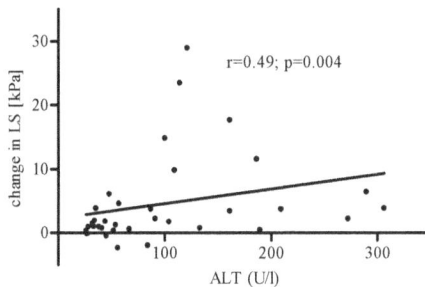

Figure 4. Correlation (Spearman's rank correlation coefficient) between ALT activity at baseline and changes in LS between baseline and FU96. ALT—alanine aminotransferase; LS—liver stiffness; kPa—kilopascal.

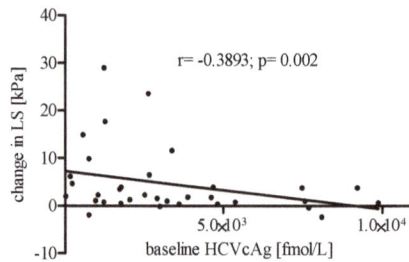

Figure 5. Correlation (Spearman's rank correlation coefficient) between baseline HCVcAg levels and change in liver stiffness between baseline and FU96. HCVcAg—HCV core antigen; kPa—kilopascal; LS—liver stiffness; fmol—femtomoles.

4. Discussion

The first descriptions of the elastography technique come from the mid-1990s [29,30]. Since then, in laboratories around the world, there has been a rapid development of this method, adding new quality to the imaging studies used so far. This technique, in a way that is easy to perform and interpret, allows one to define the "hardness" of the tissue. In a sense, it can be said that this method replaces a physical examination performed inside the human body, differentiating tissues that are healthy or pathologically changed according to their "hardness" [29]. This method is non-invasive and not time-consuming, as compared to a liver biopsy, and it is therefore easy to repeat frequently. There are some limitations in which the severity of liver inflammation and portal hypertension are the main influence on the results [31–34].

Currently, the measurement of liver stiffness is recommended by many hepatologic scientific societies as a method to determine the severity of liver disease before and after HCV treatment [8,26].

In our study, all patients had an elastographic examination performed at predetermined time points, showing a total reduction in stiffness in the vast majority of patients. This observation has already been made in earlier studies [35–39]. In our cohort, the range of changes in kPa was −4.2 to 41.8 kPa between baseline and FU24, 2.3 kPa to 29 kPa between baseline and FU96, and −2.6 to 18.7 between EOT and FU96.

According to the results of some previous studies, we have demonstrated that patients undergoing effective HCV treatment lower their LS values during follow-up (in FU24 by 1.1 kPa) and long-term observation (in FU96 by 2 kPa) in relation to baseline. In the Arima et al. study, patients treated with pegylated interferon (pegIFN) and RBV were followed, observing a mean LS drop by 5.3 (4.1–6.3) kPa in two-year follow-up [37]. However, in the Hezode et al. study, the median decrease compared to baseline at the end of follow-up was 3.4 kPa, vs. 1.8 kPa in the patients who did not achieve an SVR [38]. Due to the 100% effectiveness of treatment in our cohort, we were unable to determine such a relationship. In the ANRS CO13 HEPAVIH Cohort study, patients with HIV/HCV co-therapy remaining on two- or three-drug therapy (pegINF plus RBV with or without protease inhibitor) were investigated [39]. It was observed that achieving SVR is an independent predictor of obtaining an LS decrease. For LS evaluation, the transient elastography method was used in the studies described above and, according our knowledge, there are insufficient trials in which the SWE method was used in patients with antiviral treatment. In the Tada et al. study, the results of 210 patients treated with daclatasvir and asunaprevir were analyzed, and it was found that the average LS decreased by 1.4 kPa between baseline and EOT and 2.6 kPa between baseline and FU24, which is consistent with our results [40]. It should be noted that the type of DAA regimen used made no difference.

We also found that a significant decrease in LS occurred during both periods, antiviral therapy (between baseline and EOT $p = 0.008$) and in the long-term follow-up (between EOT and FU96 $p = 0.0002$; between FU24 and FU96 $p = 0.005$) as well. In the previously mentioned Arima et al. study and the

Chekuri et al. study, no further decrease in LS was observed after treatment in long-term follow-up—no change between in LS between 1 and 2 years of follow-up [35,37]. Conversely, in the Tada et al. study, as mentioned above, an LS decrease was also observed 24 weeks after therapy completion [40]. In the Taachi et al. trial in patients undergoing simeprevir combined with pegINF and RBV, similar results were obtained (after FU24 LS decreased by 14%) using the acoustic radiation force impulse elastography technique [41]. It can be hypothesized that the differences were influenced by the applied treatment (pegINF vs non-interferon therapies) and the method used to measure LS. The effect on the above results in our study may be due to the relatively high percentage of patients with liver cirrhosis, as well.

In our study, statistically significant changes in LS were observed in patients with more advanced liver fibrosis at F3 and F4 (p = 0.02 and 0.0004 respectively). Higher levels of liver stiffness before treatment and greater LS reduction after treatment in treatment experienced patients was related to more advanced disease in this population compared to treatment naïve. In previous studies, in patients treated with pegIFN in whom fibrosis was evaluated by liver biopsy, fibrotic regression was observed in long-term observation [42–45]. In these studies, fibrosis declined by 29–82% depending on the time of observation (from 1.6 to 5.2 years). In the Arima et al. study it was found that in 76% of patients who had F3–F4 fibrosis by liver biopsy prior to treatment, deduced fibrosis was reduced by 2 points in the fibrotic scale, and 46% of these patients had a reduction in fibrosis to F0–F1 (measured LS after treatment) [37]. It can be assumed that the LS changes not only illustrate the decline of the inflammatory process in the liver but also the regression of fibrosis and the LS measurement can visualize it in a faster way than the liver biopsy.

In previous studies, it has already been confirmed that as a result of antiviral treatment, there is an improvement in some parameters that assess liver function. In the Miyaki et al. study, they found that in patients who achieved SVR, a reduction in the AFP level, ALT activity, and platelet count were observed [46]. In a larger group of patients, in a more detailed analysis, this observation was confirmed by Tada et al. [40]. In our group of patients, we found improvement in albumin and ALT levels. However, the level of platelets did not change significantly, which is in contrast to some of the previous studies [35,40]. Probably due to the transient hyperbilirubinemia associated with the treatment (OMB/PRV/rtv ± DSV ± RBV), a statistically significant decrease in the level of bilirubin between baseline and FU24 and FU96 was observed. A similar decrease in bilirubin was observed by Deterding et al. [47]. One of the limitations of elastography is the effect on aminotransferase activity, or severity of inflammation. In our study we found that patients with advanced inflammation and ALT above 100 U/L had a statistically greater LS change between baseline and FU96, which is consistent with previous studies [40,47,48]. We also found, similarly to Chekuri et al., a positive correlation between the size of LS change and ALT activity between baseline and FU96 [35].

HCV is a well-known viral carcinogen, causing a high risk of HCC development in the infected liver. A well-established marker of this type of cancer is AFP. In our study, the elevated level of AFP at baseline indicates in most patients the presence of inflammation and necrotic processes in the liver and the accompanying processes of parenchymal reconstruction related to advanced fibrosis. During the follow-up at the end of treatment there was a statistically significant decrease in AFP concentration compared to baseline during EOT from −0.96 to 88.35 ng/dL, and during FU24 from −2.26 to 89.31 ng/dL. It should be noted that the concentration of AFP stabilized in the period between FU24 and FU96.

We did not find any statistically significant differences in the BMI index. In various studies, the results are ambiguous. Chekuri et al. observed a statistically significant increase in BMI, while in the study by Patton et al. there was no such relationship [35,49]. Chekuri et al. as the reason for the increase in BMI suggested hypermetabolism related to reduction of HCV associated inflammation, but this finding requires further studies.

To the best of our knowledge, this is the first study to evaluate the correlation between HCV core antigen and changes in liver stiffness during anti-viral treatment. The main advantage of HCVcAg is its excellent correlation with HCV RNA accompanied by much lower costs [50–52]. In our previous study baseline HCVcAg concentration correlated with HCV RNA level, its on-treatment decline was faster, and it predicted a virologic response [7].

In our study, all patients achieved an SSR, i.e., HCVcAg was undetectable at the end of treatment and this effect was maintained during a six-month follow-up. We also found a statistically significant negative correlation between changes in LS between baseline and FU96 and baseline HCVcAg. Considering that the level of LS changes depends on the severity of inflammation (ALT), a lower concentration of HCVcAg may allow an increased inflammatory response and therefore changes in LS are bigger. However, the importance of this correlation requires further research on a larger group of patients.

The advantage of our study is its prospective nature, its innovation in the assessment of changes in liver stiffness and the applied treatment based on DAA regimens. Additionally, for the first time, we analyzed the impact of HCVcAg changes on liver stiffness during antiviral treatment.

One of the most important limitations of our work is the relatively small group of patients and the lack of comparative results of liver biopsies through which a more detailed analysis could be carried out, but it could be currently questionable from the ethical point of view due to the availability of non-invasive methods of liver evaluation. Moreover, due to excellent antiviral efficacy of DAA therapy, we were not able to compare LS dynamics in responders and non-responders.

5. Conclusions

We demonstrated that liver stiffness measured with shear wave elastography significantly declined during and after treatment of chronic hepatitis C infection with direct acting antivirals. It was accompanied by improvement in some liver function measures, and the disappearance of both HCV core antigen and RNA.

Acknowledgments: This study was partially funded by a grant from Medical University of Bialystok in Poland, grant number N/ST/ZB/15/001/1156 (153-56 834L). Covering the costs to publish in open access was funded by foundation "Medycyna Podróży" Bialystok, Poland.

Author Contributions: Both authors contributed to the article equally.

Conflicts of Interest: Mariusz Łucejko has served as a speaker Gilead, Merck. Robert Flisiak has served as a speaker and an advisory board member for AbbVie, Gilead, Janssen, Merck and Roche.

References

1. Blach, S.; Zeuzem, S.; Manns, M. Polaris Observatory HCV Collaborators. Global prevalence and genotype distribution of hepatitis C virus infection in 2015: A modelling study. *Lancet Gastroenterol. Hepatol.* **2017**, *2*, 161–176. [CrossRef]
2. Alkhouri, N.; Lawitz, E.; Poordad, F. Novel treatments for chronic hepatitis C: Closing the remaining gaps. *Curr. Opin. Pharmacol.* **2017**, *37*, 107–111. [CrossRef] [PubMed]
3. Morgan, J.R.; Servidone, M.; Easterbrook, P.; Linas, B.P. Economic evaluation of HCV testing approaches in low and middle income countries. *BMC Infect. Dis.* **2017**, *17* (Suppl. 1), 697. [CrossRef] [PubMed]
4. Jülicher, P.; Galli, C. Identifying cost-effective screening algorithms for active hepatitis C virus infections in a high prevalence setting. *J. Med. Econ.* **2017**, *7*, 1–10. [CrossRef] [PubMed]
5. Hullegie, S.J.; GeurtsvanKessel, C.H.; Van der Eijk, A.A.; Ramakers, C.; Rijnders, B.J.A. HCV antigen instead of RNA testing to diagnose acute HCV in patients treated in the Dutch Acute HCV in HIV Study. *J. Int. AIDS* **2017**, *20*, 21621. [CrossRef] [PubMed]
6. Duchesne, L.; Njouom, R.; Lissock, F.; Tamko-Mella, G.F.; Rallier, S.; Poiteau, L.; Soulier, A.; Chevaliez, S.; Vernet, G.; Rouveau, N.; et al. HCV Ag quantification as a one-step procedure in diagnosing chronic hepatitis C infection in Cameroon: The ANRS 12336 study. *J. Int. AIDS Soc.* **2017**, *20*, 21446. [CrossRef] [PubMed]
7. Łucejko, M.; Flisiak, R. Quantitative measurement of HCV core antigen for management of interferon-free therapy in HCV infected patients. *Antivir. Ther.* **2017**. [CrossRef] [PubMed]
8. European Association for the Study of the Liver. Recommendations on Treatment of Hepatitis C 2016. *J. Hepatol.* **2017**, *66*, 153–194. [CrossRef]

9. Bravo, A.A.; Sheth, S.G.; Chopra, S. Liver biopsy. *N. Engl. J. Med.* **2001**, *344*, 495–500. [CrossRef] [PubMed]

10. The French METAVIR Cooperative Study Group. Intraobserver and interobserver variations in liver biopsy interpretation in patients with chronic hepatitis C. *Hepatology* **1994**, *20*, 15–20.

11. Bedossa, P.; Dargere, D.; Paradis, V. Sampling variability of liver fibrosis in chronic hepatitis C. *Hepatology* **2003**, *38*, 1449–1457. [CrossRef] [PubMed]

12. Piccinino, F.; Sagnelli, E.; Pasquale, G.; Giusti, G. Complications following percutaneous liver biopsy. A multicentre retrospective study on 68,276 biopsies. *J. Hepatol.* **1986**, *2*, 165–173. [CrossRef]

13. Friedrich-Rust, M.; Poynard, T.; Castera, L. Critical comparison of elastography methods to assess chronic liver disease. *Nat. Rev. Gastroenterol. Hepatol.* **2016**, *13*, 402–411. [CrossRef] [PubMed]

14. Castera, L.; Chan, H.L.Y.; Arrese, M.; The Clinical Practice Guideline Panel. EASL-ALEH clinical practice guidelines: Noninvasive tests for evaluation of liver disease severity and prognosis. *J. Hepatol.* **2015**, *63*, 237–264.

15. Sandrin, L.; Fourquet, B.; Hasquenoph, J.M. Transient elastography: A new noninvasive method for assessment of hepatic fibrosis. *Ultrasound Med. Biol.* **2003**, *29*, 1705–1713. [CrossRef] [PubMed]

16. Bercoff, J.; Tanter, M.; Fink, M. Supersonic shear imaging: A new technique for soft tissue elasticity mapping. *IEEE Trans. Ultrason. Ferroelectr. Freq. Control* **2004**, *51*, 396–409. [CrossRef] [PubMed]

17. Bavu, E.; Gennisson, J.-L.; Couade, M.; Bercoff, J.; Mallet, V.; Fink, M.; Badel, A.; Vallet-Pichard, A.; Nalpas, B.; Tanter, M.; et al. Noninvasive in vivo liver fibrosis evaluation using supersonic shear imaging: A clinical study on 113 hepatitis C virus patients. *Ultrasound Med. Biol.* **2011**, *37*, 1361–1373. [CrossRef] [PubMed]

18. Tsochatzis, E.A.; Gurusamy, K.S.; Ntaoula, S.; Cholongitas, E.; Davidson, B.R.; Burroughs, A.K. Elastography for the diagnosis of severity of fibrosis in chronic liver disease: A meta-analysis of diagnostic accuracy. *J. Hepatol.* **2011**, *54*, 650–659. [CrossRef] [PubMed]

19. Deffieux, T.; Gennisson, J.L.; Bousquet, L.; Corouge, M.; Cosconea, S.; Amroun, D.; Tripon, S.; Terris, B.; Mallet, V.; Sogni, P.; et al. Investigating liver stiffness and viscosity for fibrosis, steatosis and activity staging using shear wave elastography. *J. Hepatol.* **2015**, *62*, 317–324. [CrossRef] [PubMed]

20. Ogasawara, N.; Kobayashi, M.; Akuta, N.; Kominami, Y.; Fujiyama, S.; Kawamura, Y.; Sezaki, H.; Hosaka, T.; Suzuki, F.; Saitoh, S.; et al. Serial changes in liver stiffness and controlled attenuation parameter following direct-acting antiviral therapy against hepatitis C virus genotype 1b. *J. Med. Virol.* **2018**, *90*, 313–331. [CrossRef] [PubMed]

21. Elsharkawy, A.; Alem, S.A.; Fouad, R.; El Raziky, M.; El Akel, W.; Abdo, M.; Tantawi, O.; AbdAllah, M.; Bourliere, M.; Esmat, G. Changes in liver stiffness measurements and fibrosis scores following sofosbuvir based treatment regimens without interferon. *J. Gastroenterol. Hepatol.* **2017**, *32*, 1624–1630. [CrossRef] [PubMed]

22. Cassinotto, C.; Lapuyade, B.; Mouries, A.; Hiriart, J.B.; Vergniol, J.; Gaye, D.; Castain, C.; Le Bail, B.; Chermak, F.; Foucher, J.; et al. Non-invasive assessment of liver fibrosis with impulse elastography: Comparison of supersonic shear imaging with ARFI and FibroScanVR. *J. Hepatol.* **2014**, *61*, 550–557. [CrossRef] [PubMed]

23. Guibal, A.; Renosi, G.; Rode, A.; Scoazec, J.Y.; Guillaud, O.; Chardon, L.; Munteanu, M.; Dumortier, J.; Collin, F.; Lefort, T.; et al. Shear wave elastography: An accurate technique to stage liver fibrosis in chronic liver diseases. *Diagn. Interv. Imaging* **2016**, *97*, 91–99. [CrossRef] [PubMed]

24. Sigrist, R.M.S.; Liau, J.; Kaffas, A.E.; Chammas, M.C.; Willmann, J.K. Ultrasound Elastography: Review of Techniques and Clinical Applications. *Theranostics* **2017**, *7*, 1303–1329. [CrossRef] [PubMed]

25. Flisiak, R.; Pogorzelska, J.; Berak, H.; Horban, A.; Orłowska, I.; Simon, K.; Tuchendler, E.; Madej, G.; Piekarska, A.; Jabłkowski, M.; et al. Prevalence of HCV genotypes in Poland—The EpiTer study. *Clin. Exp. Hepatol.* **2016**, *2*, 144–148. [CrossRef] [PubMed]

26. Polish Group of HCV Experts; Halota, W.; Flisiak, R.; Boroń-Kaczmarska, A.; Juszczyk, J.; Małkowski, P.; Pawłowska, M.; Simon, K.; Tomasiewicz, K. Recommendations for the treatment of hepatitis C issued by the Polish Group of HCV Experts—2016. *Clin. Exp. Hepatol.* **2016**, *2*, 27–33. [CrossRef] [PubMed]

27. Ferraioli, G.; Tinelli, C.; Dal Bello, B.; Zicchetti, M.; Filice, G.; Filice, C. Liver Fibrosis Study Group. Accuracy of real-time shear wave elastography for assessing liver fibrosis in chronic hepatitis C: A pilot study. *Hepatology* **2012**, *56*, 2125–2133. [CrossRef] [PubMed]

28. Muller, M.; Gennisson, J.-L.; Deffieux, T.; Tanter, M.; Fink, M. Quantitative viscoelasticity mapping of human liver using supersonic shear imaging: Preliminary in vivo feasibility study. *Ultrasound Med. Biol.* **2009**, *35*, 219–229. [CrossRef] [PubMed]

29. Sarvazyan, A.P. A new approach to remote ultrasonic evaluation of viscoelastic properties of tissues for diagnostics and healing monitoring. In Proceedings of the ARPA/ONR Medical Ultrasonic Imaging Technology Workshop, Landsdowne, VA, USA, 24–26 January 1995.

30. Rudenko, O.V.; Sarvazyan, A.P.; Emelianov, S.Y. Acoustic radiation force and streaming induced by focused nonlinear ultrasound in a dissipative medium. *J. Acoust. Soc. Am.* **1996**, *99*, 2791–2798. [CrossRef]

31. Poynard, T.; Pham, T.; Perazzo, H.; Munteanu, M.; Luckina, E.; Elaribi, D.; Ngo, Y.; Bonyhay, L.; Seurat, N.; Legroux, M.; et al. Real-Time Shear Wave versus Transient Elastography for Predicting Fibrosis: Applicability, and Impact of Inflammation and Steatosis. A Non-Invasive Comparison. *PLoS ONE* **2016**, *11*, e0163276. [CrossRef] [PubMed]

32. Yoon, K.T.; Lim, S.M.; Park, J.Y.; Kim, D.Y.; Ahn, S.H.; Han, K.H.; Chon, C.Y.; Cho, M.; Lee, J.W.; Kim, S.U. Liver stiffness measurement using acoustic radiation force impulse (ARFI) elastography and effect of necroinflammation. *Dig. Dis. Sci.* **2012**, *57*, 1682–1691. [CrossRef] [PubMed]

33. Arena, U.; Vizzutti, F.; Corti, G.; Ambu, S.; Stasi, C.; Bresci, S.; Moscarella, S.; Boddi, V.; Petrarca, A.; Laffi, G.; et al. Acute viral hepatitis increases liver stiffness values measured by transient elastography. *Hepatology* **2008**, *47*, 380–384. [CrossRef] [PubMed]

34. Coco, B.; Oliveri, F.; Maina, A.M.; Ciccorossi, P.; Sacco, R.; Colombatto, P.; Bonino, F.; Brunetto, M.R. Transient elastography: A new surrogate marker of liver fibrosis influenced by major changes of transaminases. *J. Viral Hepat.* **2007**, *14*, 360–369. [CrossRef] [PubMed]

35. Chekuri, S.; Nickerson, J.; Bichoupan, K.; Sefcik, R.; Doobay, K.; Chang, S.; DelBello, D.; Harty, A.; Dieterich, D.T.; Perumalswami, P.V.; et al. Liver Stiffness Decreases Rapidly in Response to Successful Hepatitis C Treatment and Then Plateaus. *PLoS ONE* **2016**, *11*, e0159413. [CrossRef] [PubMed]

36. Wang, J.H.; Changchien, C.S.; Hung, C.H.; Tung, W.C.; Kee, K.M.; Chen, C.H.; Hu, T.H.; Lee, C.M.; Lu, S.N. Liver stiffness decrease after effective antiviral therapy in patients with chronic hepatitis C: Longitudinal study using FibroScan. *J. Gastroenterol. Hepatol.* **2010**, *25*, 964–969. [CrossRef] [PubMed]

37. Arima, Y.; Kawabe, N.; Hashimoto, S.; Harata, M.; Nitta, Y.; Murao, M.; Nakano, T.; Shimazaki, H.; Kobayashi, K.; Ichino, N.; et al. Reduction of liver stiffness by interferon treatment in the patients with chronic hepatitis, C. *Hepatol. Res.* **2010**, *40*, 383–392. [CrossRef] [PubMed]

38. Hezode, C.; Castera, L.; Roudot-Thoraval, F.; Bouvier-Alias, M.; Rosa, I.; Roulot, D.; Leroy, V.; Mallat, A.; Pawlotsky, J.M. Liver stiffness diminishes with antiviral response in chronic hepatitis, C. *Aliment. Pharmacol. Ther.* **2011**, *34*, 656–663. [CrossRef] [PubMed]

39. ANRS CO13 HEPAVIH Cohort. Regression of liver stiffness after sustained hepatitis C virus (HCV) virological responses among HIV/HCV—Coinfected patients. *Aids* **2015**, *29*, 1821–1830. [CrossRef]

40. Tada, T.; Kumada, T.; Toyoda, H.; Mizuno, K.; Sone, Y.; Kataoka, S.; Hashinokuchi, S. Improvement of liver stiffness in patients with hepatitis C virus infection who received direct-acting antiviral therapy and achieved sustained virological response. *J. Gastroenterol. Hepatol.* **2017**, *32*, 198–1988. [CrossRef] [PubMed]

41. Tachi, Y.; Hirai, T.; Kojima, Y.; Ishizu, Y.; Honda, T.; Kuzuya, T.; Hayashi, K.; Ishigami, M.; Goto, H. Liver stiffness reduction correlates with histological characteristics of hepatitis C patients with sustained virological response. *Liver Int.* **2017**. [CrossRef] [PubMed]

42. Shiratori, Y.; Imazeki, F.; Moriyama, M.; Yano, M.; Arakawa, Y.; Yokosuka, O.; Kuroki, T.; Nishiguchi, S.; Sata, M.; Yamada, G.; et al. Histologic improvement of fibrosis in patients with hepatitis C who have sustained response to interferon therapy. *Ann. Intern. Med.* **2000**, *132*, 517–524. [CrossRef] [PubMed]

43. Veldt, B.J.; Saracco, G.; Boyer, N.; Cammà, C.; Bellobuono, A.; Hopf, U.; Castillo, I.; Weiland, O.; Nevens, F.; Hansen, B.E.; et al. Long term clinical outcome of chronic hepatitis C patients with sustained virological response to interferon monotherapy. *Gut* **2004**, *53*, 1504–1508. [CrossRef] [PubMed]

44. Toccaceli, F.; Laghi, V.; Capurso, L.; Koch, M.; Sereno, S.; Scuderi, M. Long-term liver histology improvement in patients with chronic hepatitis C and sustained response to interferon. *J. Viral Hepat.* **2003**, *10*, 126–133. [CrossRef] [PubMed]

45. George, S.L.; Bacon, B.R.; Brunt, E.M.; Mihindukulasuriya, K.L.; Hoffmann, J.; Di Bisceglie, A.M. Clinical, virologic, histologic, and biochemical outcomes after successful HCV therapy: A 5-year follow-up of 150 patients. *Hepatology* **2009**, *49*, 729–738. [CrossRef] [PubMed]

46. Miyaki, E.; Imamura, M.; Hiraga, N.; Murakami, E.; Kawaoka, T.; Tsuge, M.; Hiramatsu, A.; Kawakami, Y.; Aikata, H.; Hayes, C.N.; et al. Daclatasvir and asunaprevir treatment improves liver function parameters and reduces liver fibrosis markers in chronic hepatitis C patients. *Hepatol. Res.* **2016**, *46*, 758–764. [CrossRef] [PubMed]

47. Deterding, K.; Honer Zu Siederdissen, C.; Port, K.; Solbach, P.; Sollik, L.; Kirschner, J.; Mix, C.; Cornberg, J.; Worzala, D.; Mix, H.; et al. Improvement of liver function parameters in advanced HCV-associated liver cirrhosis by IFN-free antiviral therapies. *Aliment. Pharmacol. Ther.* **2015**, *42*, 889–901. [CrossRef] [PubMed]

48. Tachi, Y.; Hirai, T.; Ishizu, Y.; Honda, T.; Kuzuya, T.; Hayashi, K.; Ishigami, M.; Goto, H. α-fetoprotein levels after interferon therapy predict regression of liver fibrosis in patients with sustained virological response. *J. Gastroenterol. Hepatol.* **2016**, *31*, 1001–1008. [CrossRef] [PubMed]

49. Patton, H.M.; Patel, K.; Behling, C.; Bylund, D.; Blatt, L.M.; Vallee, M.; Heaton, S.; Conrad, A.; Pockros, P.J.; McHutchison, J.G.; et al. The impact of steatosis on disease progression and early and sustained treatment response in chronic hepatitis C patients. *J. Hepatol.* **2004**, *40*, 484–490. [CrossRef] [PubMed]

50. Aoyagi, K.; Ohue, C.; Iida, K.; Kimura, T.; Tanaka, E.; Kiyosawa, K.; Yagi, S. Development of a simple and highly sensitive enzyme immunoassay for hepatitis C virus core antigen. *J. Clin. Microbiol.* **1999**, *37*, 1802–1808. [PubMed]

51. Mederacke, I.; Potthoff, A.; Meyer-Olson, D.; Meier, M.; Raupach, R.; Manns, M.P.; Wedemeyer, H.; Tillmann, H.L. HCV core antigen testing in HIV- and HBV-coinfected patients, and in HCV-infected patients on hemodialysis. *J. Clin. Virol.* **2012**, *53*, 110–115. [CrossRef] [PubMed]

52. Łucejko, M.; Grzeszczuk, A.; Jaroszewicz, J.; Flisiak, R. Serum HCV core antigen concentration in HCV monoinfection and HCV/HIV coinfection. *Pol. Merkur. Lekarski* **2013**, *35*, 72–76. [PubMed]

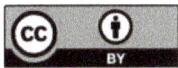

© 2018 by the authors. Licensee MDPI, Basel, Switzerland. This article is an open access article distributed under the terms and conditions of the Creative Commons Attribution (CC BY) license (http://creativecommons.org/licenses/by/4.0/).

applied
sciences

MDPI

Article

Non-Invasive Assessment of Hepatic Fibrosis by Elastic Measurement of Liver Using Magnetic Resonance Tagging Images

Xuejun Zhang [1,3,]*, **Xiangrong Zhou [2], Takeshi Hara [2] and Hiroshi Fujita [2]**

[1] School of Computer and Electronic Information, Guangxi University, Nanning 530004, Guangxi, China
[2] Department of Electrical, Electronic and Computer Engineering, Gifu University, Gifu 501-1193, Japan; zxr@fjt.info.gifu-u.ac.jp (X.Z.); hara@fjt.info.gifu-u.ac.jp (T.H.); fujita@info.gifu-u.ac.jp (H.F.)
[3] Guangxi Key Laboratory of Multimedia Communications and Network Technology, Nanning 530004, Guangxi, China
*   Correspondence: xjzhang@gxu.edu.cn; Tel.: +86-771-323-6216

Received: 11 February 2018; Accepted: 7 March 2018; Published: 14 March 2018

Abstract: To date, the measurement of the stiffness of liver requires a special vibrational tool that limits its application in many hospitals. In this study, we developed a novel method for automatically assessing the elasticity of the liver without any use of contrast agents or mechanical devices. By calculating the non-rigid deformation of the liver from magnetic resonance (MR) tagging images, the stiffness was quantified as the displacement of grids on the liver image during a forced exhalation cycle. Our methods include two major processes: (1) quantification of the non-rigid deformation as the bending energy (BE) based on the thin-plate spline method in the spatial domain and (2) calculation of the difference in the power spectrum from the tagging images, by using fast Fourier transform in the frequency domain. By considering 34 cases (17 normal and 17 abnormal liver cases), a remarkable difference between the two groups was found by both methods. The elasticity of the liver was finally analyzed by combining the bending energy and power spectral features obtained through MR tagging images. The result showed that only one abnormal case was misclassified in our dataset, which implied our method for non-invasive assessment of liver fibrosis has the potential to reduce the traditional liver biopsy.

Keywords: computer-aided diagnosis (CAD); magnetic resonance imaging; cine-tagging; liver fibrosis; elastography; bending energy; power spectrum

---

1. Introduction

Chronic liver disease is a worldwide health problem and increases the risk of hepatic complications such as hepatocellular carcinoma (HCC) and liver failure [1]. Cirrhosis of the liver is a late stage of progressive liver disease defined as structural distortion of the entire liver by fibrosis and parenchymal nodules. The assessment of cirrhosis and chronic hepatitis highly depends on the degree of hepatic fibrosis, which is regarded as an important predictive indicator of cirrhosis [2]. As HCC is one of the most common malignancies in patients affected by these diseases [3], early detection and accurate staging of cirrhosis is an important issue in practical radiology. Generally, fibrosis is interpreted on Computed Tomography (CT) or magnetic resonance imaging (MRI) images by referring to changes in hepatic morphology, texture pattern, and the degree of liver stiffness. Although there is no effective treatment for decompensate or advanced cirrhosis, appropriate treatment such as interferon therapy is sometimes beneficial for early cirrhosis associated with viral hepatitis because fibrosis is potentially a reversible process in the early stages.

Liver biopsy, which is an effective way of measuring changes in fibrosis staging, is regarded as the gold standard for assessing, by referring to the micrograph of a liver core needle biopsy, the severity of liver disease and monitoring treatment. However, it is an invasive procedure, and significant bleeding occurs in 1–2 out of 100 patients, and it is possible to cause pain in 30–40% of cases, pneumothorax (3‰), or even death (2/10,000) [4,5]. The accuracy may also be questioned because of side effects, punctured sampling, and interobserver variability in the determination of semiquantitative fibrosis scores [6–8]. In order to decrease the need of painful biopsies, non-invasive tests using MR and ultrasound modalities have been widely used with the development of high-speed imaging devices. Recently, radiological assessments of hepatic fibrosis by magnetic resonance elastography (MRE) [8–10], gadolinium- or superparamagnetic iron-oxide-enhanced MR imaging [11,12], diffusion-weighted MR imaging [13], and real-time ultrasonographic elastography [14] have been reported. Wang et al. [15] proposed a real-time elastography for diffuse histological lesions, showing a new and promising quantitative technology for assessing liver fibrosis in patients with chronic hepatitis B using a solography-based non-invasive method. Although such new imaging technologies have greatly impacted the traditional diagnostic methods, the interpretation of the numerous diseases from different types of medical images is a tough work, especially for the inexperienced residents or general radiologists. In the last decade, different types of computer-aided detection/diagnosis (CAD) systems have been developed to ease the workload of radiologists. Some CAD systems for quantitative assessment of liver fibrosis have been shown their promising results by analyzing morphology changes [16,17] and the texture pattern of fibrosis [18] on CT/MR images. Recently, the degree of stiffness has also been analyzed through MR elastography. Muthupillai et al. [8] first proposed the method of MRE by direct visualization of propagating acoustic strain waves, and Rouvière et al. [9] then proved its usefulness. However, both ultrasonographic elastography and the above-mentioned MRE methods require special equipment, which limits their application in many hospitals.

The fibrogenic change in stiffness of the liver from soft to hard indicates a change in the liver status from normal to chronic hepatitis, to cirrhosis, and even to liver cancer. However, obtaining the physical properties of the liver, such as tissue stiffness, is not possible with traditional MR imaging technology. We preliminarily reported a novel method to measure the liver elasticity using an MR device to measure hepatic deformation and attempted to quantify the stiffness of the liver with cine-tagging MR imaging at 3T and bending energy (BE) analysis for the evaluation of hepatic fibrosis [19]. In comparison with MRE or the ultrasound elastography method, our proposed method measures the stiffness of the liver by tracking the dynamic changes in the configuration of the grid pattern and analyzing the deformation of the liver only with the MR image, without using any additional physical vibration devices. Some studies have analyzed the movement of organs or tissue of the human body (such as the heart), and measurement of the stiffness of the internal organs using an MR tagging image [20–24], but there are no reports on the liver. Although our preliminary results showed a significant difference between normal and abnormal groups, there were some overlaps of stiffness in the normal and intermediate fibrosis stages, and the number of cases in the experiment was small. Furthermore, manual input of landmarks (LMs) for calculating the BE value on each grid was rather time-consuming. In this study, a power-spectrum-based method is proposed to improve the efficiency in distinguishing normal liver tissue from abnormal liver tissue quantitatively. A combination of processing in the frequency domain with that in the spatial domain is also discussed.

2. Experimental Materials

All MR images were scanned by a 3-T superconducting system (Intera Achieva Quasar Dual; Philips Medical Systems, Eindhoven, The Netherlands) with a six-channel torso array coil. A modified spatial modulation of magnetization (SPAMM) sequence with a train of non-selective radiofrequency (RF) pulses was employed [19], after which the single-section cine MR imaging with a two-dimensional (2D) single-shot turbo field-echo sequence (repetition time(TR)/echo time(TE), 2.2/1.0 ms; flip angle, 10°; field of view, 45 × 36 cm^2; number of echo trains, 35; interpolated imaging matrix, 256 × 256; parallel imaging factor, 2; slice thickness, 10 mm; scan frequency, nine images per second) was conducted as shown in Figure 1. Cine-tagging grids with 12, 16, 20 and 24 mm stripe spacings were scanned separately in the sagittal and coronal imaging planes. We set the sagittal grids in the right hepatic lobe, so the sagittal plane did not include the heart or the porta hepatis, and the cross-sectional area of the liver was as large as possible; typically, the sagittal plane was set at the top of the right hemidiaphragm. On the other hand, we set the coronal grids in the liver, so the coronal plane included the right and left hepatic lobes as broadly as possible—typically at a ventral one-third of the entire anteroposterior dimension of the liver. MRI obtained by the cine-tagging method using the above parameters is defined as "MR tagging images" in this paper. MR tagging images used in this study were a set of sequenced images consisting of nine frames scanned per breathing cycle. It is obvious that tag grids appear clearest in the first frame (Frame 1) because it is generated at the time of inhalation, and the tag becomes gradually faded with progression to the last frame (Frame 9).

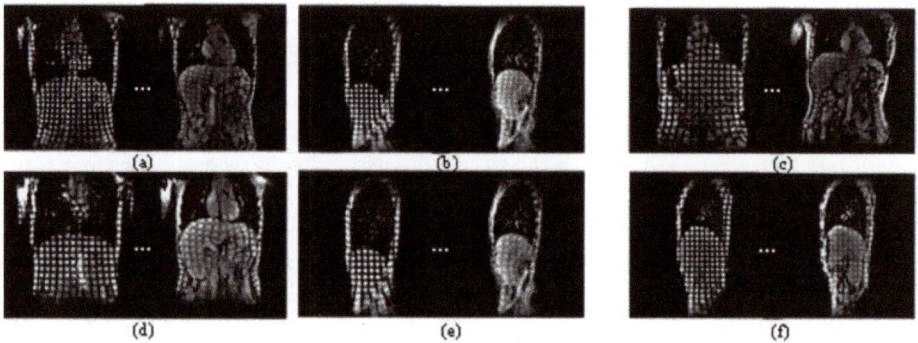

Figure 1. magnetic resonance (MR) tagging images of a healthy liver (F0) at the maximal inspiratory (frame1, left) phase and the maximal expiratory (Frame 9, right) phase, using 16 mm coronal (**a**); 16 mm sagittal (**b**); 20 mm coronal (**c**); and 20 mm sagittal (**d**) grids. For comparison; (**e**,**f**) are the images of a cirrhotic liver (F4) using 20 mm coronal and 16 mm sagittal grids, respectively. Note that the grid is deformed over 1 s of forced exhalation, and the deformation of the healthy liver is greater than that of the cirrhotic liver, which reflects the firmness of the parenchyma.

Thirty-four cases acquired from Gifu University Hospital in Japan were used in our experiment. This study was approved by the institutional review board at Gifu University, and informed consent was obtained from all patients. Out of the 34 cases, 17 were normal liver cases, and the other 17 were abnormal liver cases (6 chronic hepatitis cases and 11 liver cirrhosis cases).

3. Methods

The changing configuration of the grid pattern during forced exhalation reflects the local motion, rotation, deformation, or distortion of the liver parenchyma. The rigid transformation of tags only indicates the location of changes in the liver, not including any feature for warping measurement, which is correlated to the stiffness of the liver. Our methods for quantifying non-rigid deformation include two major processes: (1) calculation of the BE based on the thin-plate spline (TPS) method [25] in the spatial domain and (2) calculation of the difference in the power spectral values of the tags obtained by fast Fourier transform (FFT) in the frequency domain.

3.1. Calculation of Bending Energy Based on Thin-Plate Spline (TPS) Method in the Spatial Domain

The LMs indicated as yellow points in Figure 2 were placed by an experienced radiologist (W. H.) with three years of experience in MR imaging diagnosis of abdomens. Although this manual operation may be replaced by automatic methods, such as Hough transformation used in our preliminary research [26], we planned to use these gold standards in an ideal condition to accurately evaluate the performance of our methods. Figure 2 shows the coordinates of intersecting points of grids determined on (a) the first frame (before warping) and the corresponding points on (b) the last frame (after warping). The reason for setting an LM at the time of inhalation versus the time of expiration is that the difference in the strength of deformation between the normal liver and the abnormal liver conspicuously varies when the BE value is calculated when the volume of deformation of the liver is the largest. These coordinate values are processed to quantify the degree of distortion or deformation of the liver parenchyma.

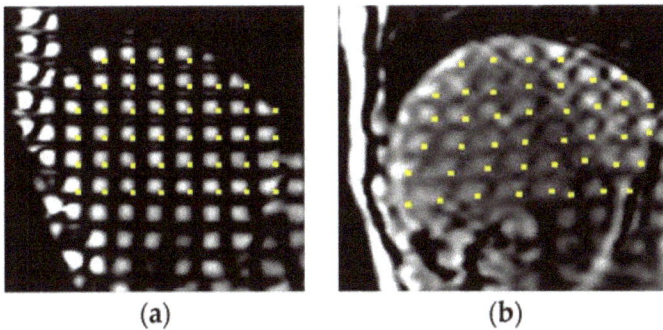

(a)   (b)

Figure 2. Landmarks (LMs) marked in yellow point were manually set by a radiologist. First, the LMs on the intersection points of grids were marked on the first frame, Frame 1 (**a**), of the MR tagging image before deformation. The corresponding LMs were then tracked and placed on the image after non-rigid transformation in the last frame, Frame 9 (**b**).

We first applied a TPS-based method referring to a physical analogy involving the bending of a thin sheet of metal, which has been well recognized and used extensively in engineering, to calculate BE values within the liver region. The TPS-based method is widely used for image transformation [25], which requires the setting of the LMs on the image before transformation and the corresponding LM transformation image.

In this study, we first set a point (x_i, y_i) as an LM on the left of the intersection point of the tag at the first frame (Figure 2a) on the MR tagging image $I(x, y)$. Then, its corresponding LM is tracked as $(x\prime_i, y\prime_i)$ at the ninth frame (Figure 2b). Here, $1 \leq i \leq n$, n is the number of LMs; $I(x\prime, y\prime)$ is an image after transformation with the TPS-based method by the mapping function $f(x, y) = [f_x(x, y), f_y(x, y)]$, which maps each point (x_i, y_i) to its homolog $(x\prime_i, y\prime_i)$. To calculate the bending energy I_f, the TPS fits the mapping function $f(x, y)$ between corresponding point-sets by minimizing the following energy function:

$$E = \iint\limits_{R^2} \left(\left(\frac{\partial^2 f}{\partial x^2}\right)^2 + 2\left(\frac{\partial^2 f}{\partial x \partial y}\right)^2 + \left(\frac{\partial^2 f}{\partial y^2}\right)^2 \right) dx dy. \tag{1}$$

There are many solutions for the function $E(x, y)$, and the I_f value is selected as the minimal value among these solutions, which satisfies the condition of $dE = 0$. The mapping function

$$f(x, y) = a_1 + a_x x + a_y y + \sum_{i=1}^{n} w_i U(|(x, y) - (x_i, y_i)|), \tag{2}$$

minimizes the energy function in Equation (3), where $U(r)$ can be defined as $U(r) = |r|$, $r = |(x, y) - (x_i, y_i)|$ is the distance between (x_i, y_i) and $(x\prime_i, y\prime_i)$, and a and w are the coefficients between $I(x, y)$ and $I(x\prime, y\prime)$, calculated as follows:

$$\begin{bmatrix} \mathbf{w} \\ \mathbf{a} \end{bmatrix} = \begin{bmatrix} \mathbf{V} \\ 0 \end{bmatrix} \begin{bmatrix} \mathbf{K} & \mathbf{P} \\ \mathbf{P}^T & 0 \end{bmatrix}^{-1}. \tag{3}$$

P, *V*, and *K* are minor determinants of *L*, where

$$P = \begin{bmatrix} 1 & x_1 & y_1 \\ 1 & x_2 & y_2 \\ \cdots & \cdots & \cdots \\ 1 & x_n & y_n \end{bmatrix}, V = \begin{bmatrix} x_1' & x_2' & \cdots & x_n' \\ y_1' & y_2' & \cdots & y_n' \end{bmatrix}, K = \begin{bmatrix} 0 & U(r_{12}) & \cdots & U(r_{1n}) \\ U(r_{21}) & 0 & \cdots & U(r_{2n}) \\ \cdots & \cdots & \cdots & \cdots \\ U(r_{n1}) & U(r_{n2}) & \cdots & 0 \end{bmatrix} \quad (4)$$

and

$$L = \begin{bmatrix} K & P \\ P^T & O \end{bmatrix}. \quad (5)$$

Based on the selected LMs on two images, the BE value of I_f is finally calculated by

$$I_f = V(L_n^{-1} K L_n^{-1}) V^T. \quad (6)$$

Therefore, the bending energy calculated by Equation (6) is regarded as the value of the non-rigid deformation of the liver. Although the TPS method is a very traditional deformation method, the use of the BE value as a classification feature is rare.

3.2. Calculation of the Difference in the Power Spectral Values of the Tags by FFT in the Frequency Domain

Manually placing the LMs is time-consuming and impractical for clinical use. To overcome this disadvantage, our method for measuring non-rigid deformation is modified to the frequency domain processing using a 2D FFT method. Because the main patterns in the MR tagging image are grids that periodically appear at a certain principal frequency f_0 (or wavelength) corresponding to the distance between the intervals of the grids; any changes in the interval of the grids will make its frequency shift from f_0 to $f_0 + \Delta f$. A larger change in the shape of the grids results in a wider distribution of the range of Δf, which represents different frequency components. Such a deformation, very similar to the optic phenomenon, appears to be lost in focus at a frequency point of f_0 on its 2D power spectrum image. This implies another way of quantifying the non-rigid deformation by applying the 2D FFT method to an MR tagging image and then comparing the difference in the power spectral values in a candidate region around f_0.

FFT is an efficient algorithm for computing the discrete Fourier transform (DFT); the calculation of the DFT on a limited dataset that greatly decreases the computing iterations and time is optimized. 2D DFT on a 256 × 256 MR tagging image can be written as

$$F(u,v) = \sum_{x=0}^{255} \sum_{y=0}^{255} F(x,y) e^{-j2\pi(xu/256 + yv/256)} \quad (7)$$

where $F(x,y)$ is the gray value at point (x,y) on an MR tagging image in the spatial domain, and $F(u,v)$ is the complex value at (u,v) corresponding to the transverse and longitudinal frequency components of $F(x,y)$ in the frequency domain derived from FFT, where $x,y,u,v \in (0,1,2,3 \cdots 256 - 1)$. j is the imaginary unit. The matrix of the power spectrum is calculated as

$$PWS_F(u,v) = |F(u,v)|^2 = Fr^2(u,v) + Fi^2(u,v) \quad (8)$$

where $PWS_F(u,v)$ is the power spectrum of $F(u,v)$, and $Fr(u,v)$ and $Fi(u,v)$ are the real and imaginary parts of $F(u,v)$, respectively. The low-frequency components (small gray-filled squares) distribute in the four corners of matrix $F(u,v)$, and the highest frequencies are located in the middle of the matrix as shown in Figure 3a. To visualize the power spectrum into a gray-scale image for further processing, we re-arrange the four quadrants from the power spectrum matrix $PWS_F(u,v)$ into $PWS_I(u,v)$ as shown in Figure 3b. Because of the symmetries of the spectrum, the entire set of quadrant positions can be diagonally replaced following the direction of the arrows indicated in Figure 3a after replacing the highest frequencies at the corners of the matrix. Because the main energy is concentrated in the low-frequency range, which could interfere with the main frequency component of f_0, logarithm transformation is applied to $PWS_I(u,v)$, and we obtain a new matrix $P(x,y)$, known as the power spectral image (PSI), which is expressed as

$$P(x,y) = \log PWS_I(u,v). \qquad (9)$$

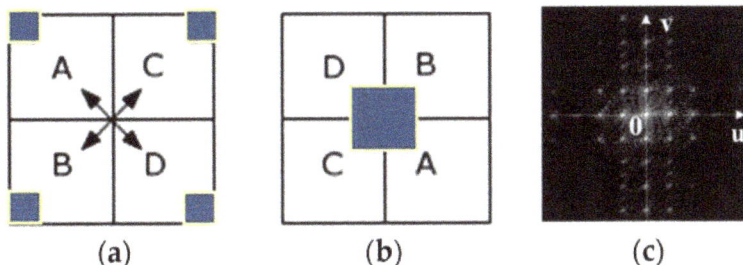

Figure 3. Discrete Fourier transform (DFT) of a 2D MR tagging image with its (a) original power spectrum; (b) frequency range replaced by a power spectrum; (c) power spectral image (PSI) after logarithm transformation.

Figure 3c indicates the structure of tags on the PSI with a typical grid pattern for the normal liver or abnormal liver on the first frame of the MR tagging image before transformation. In Figure 4, the points on the u axis are the principal frequency of the tag (Region 4) and its high harmonic components in the transverse direction, whereas points on the v axis are the principal frequency of the tag (Region 2) and its high harmonic components in the longitudinal direction. We should note that the intersectional tags in the diagonal directions also appear periodically; therefore, other points (Region 1 and Region 3) are conspicuously plotted on the PSI as well, which makes the power spectral value of the tag appear equidistantly in the frequency domain. Their corresponding power spectra are plotted using all cases (normal or abnormal) to determine the most sensitive frequency component among Regions 1–4.

To avoid the unwanted components of the power spectrum in the PSI that pertain to other organs or tissues, the liver region (bottom of Figure 5a,b) is manually segmented from the original MR tagging images (top of Figure 5a,b) beforehand. Note that the PSI has better quality with segmented liver images (bottom of Figure 5c,d) than with the original images (top of Figure 5c,d).

With the deformation of the liver, the displacement of the tag differs between the normal and abnormal livers in the spatial domain, which will also result in differences in the power spectrum in the frequency domain. It is obvious that the movement of the tags from Frame 1 to Frame 9 in the longitudinal direction (Region 4 in Figure 4) is greater than that in the transverse direction; thus, the principal frequency f_0 in the transverse direction (the right square in Figure 6a,b) is selected as a region of interest (ROI) for calculating the magnitude of the power spectrum. A larger deformation of the liver results in a larger difference in the power spectrum of the two ROIs. Therefore, the difference in the power spectral (DPS) values of the tag region between the first frame and the ninth frame of the MR tagging image in the 2D frequency domain is high on the normal liver (Figure 6a) and low on the abnormal liver (Figure 6b).

In a 5 × 5 ROI, the power spectral value in the coordinate (x,y), which has the maximum power spectral value $p_1(x,y)$, is located in the first frame of the MR tagging image, whereas the power spectral value at the same coordinate of (x,y) is $p_9(x,y)$ in the ninth frame of the MR tagging image. The DPS value between $p_1(x,y)$ and $p_9(x,y)$ is determined by $p_{1-9}(x,y) = p_1(x,y) - p_9(x,y)$.

(a)

(b)

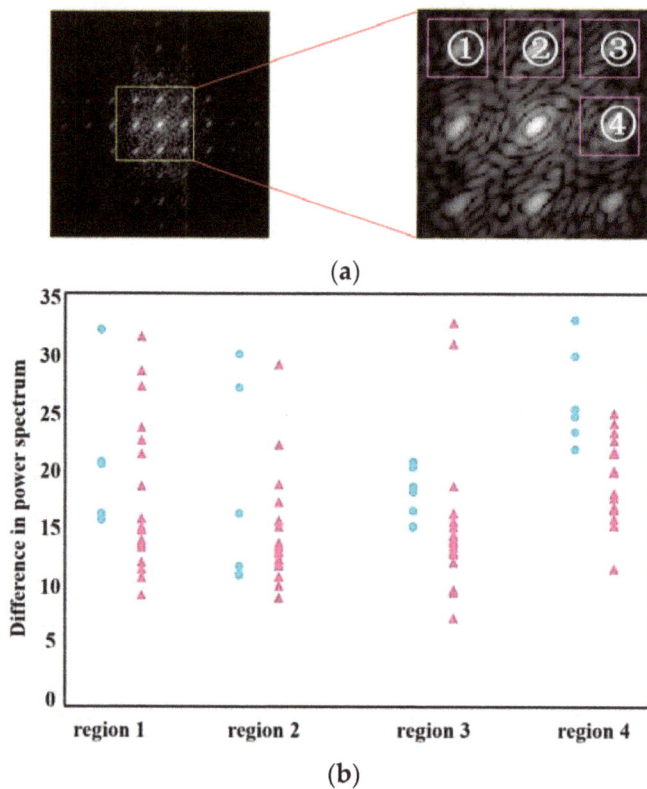

Figure 4. Four principal frequencies in four directions are marked as Regions 1–4 (**a**), and their corresponding power spectra are plotted using all the cases to determine the most sensitive frequency component (**b**) for differentiating normal cases (•) from abnormal cases (▲).

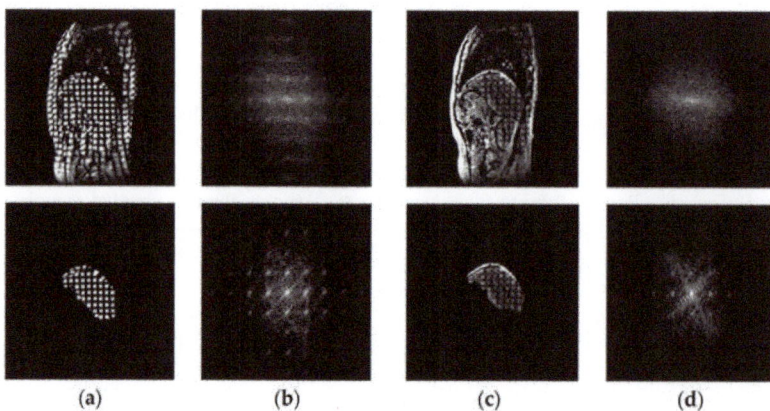

Figure 5. Segmentation of the liver region from an original MR tagging image in Frame 1 (**a**) and the corresponding PSIs (**b**); (**c**,**d**) spatial and frequency images derived from Frame 9. Note that the PSIs have better contrast in the segmented liver images (bottom) than in the original images (top).

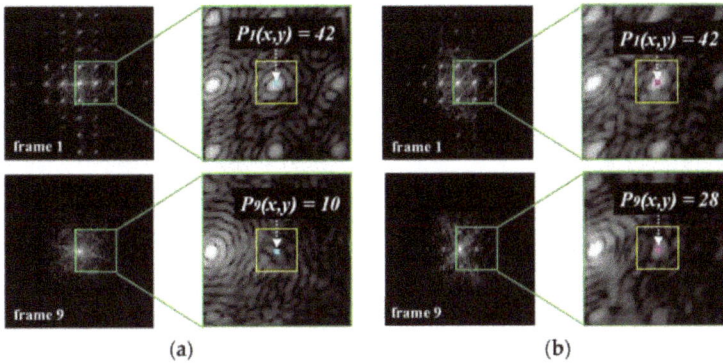

Figure 6. Difference in the power spectral (DPS) value within a 5×5 ROI between the first frame and the ninth frame of the MR tagging image in the 2D frequency domain is relatively large on the normal liver (**a**) and small on the abnormal, cirrhotic liver (**b**).

3.3. Classification Method

The self-organizing map (SOM) [27] is an excellent tool in the exploratory phase of data mining. Compared with the other traditional neural network algorithms, the SOM has the advantage of tolerating very low accuracy in the representation of its signals and synaptic weights. It projects an input space on prototypes of a low-dimensional regular grid that can be effectively used to visualize and explore properties of the data. In our study, the input vectors are the BE and DPS values, and similar units can be clustered into normal and abnormal liver groups, with parameters set as follows: size = 34; mat: [2, 2]; sigma = 0.2; maxiterator = 2000.

4. Results and Discussion

Figure 1a shows cine-tagging images using a 16 mm sagittal grid in a 56-year-old male patient with fibrosis scores equal to F0. The first image (Frame 1) obtained at the maximum inspiratory phase shows the grid without distortion. The last image (Frame 9) obtained at the maximum expiratory phase shows the grid with evident distortion. The coordinate values of a given grid intersection on the first image (x, y) and those of the corresponding grid intersection on the last image (x_i, y_i) were determined by a radiologist. The BE value calculated using these images was 2.52, and its corresponding DPS value was $p_{1-9}(x,y) = 42 - 10 = 32$, as shown in Figure 6a. Figure 1f shows a 72-year-old male patient with fibrosis scores equal to F4. The grid in the first image has no distortion, whereas the last image obtained at the maximum expiratory phase shows that the grid shifted slightly upward, but there is no distortion with the grid. The BE value calculated using these images was as low as 0.57, and its corresponding DPS value was $p_{1-9}(x,y) = 42 - 28 = 14$, as shown in Figure 6b. It is evident that the value of the non-rigid deformation is high if the value of BE/DPS is high. On the other hand, the deformation is low if the value of BE/DPS is low.

The reason for setting an LM at the time of inhalation versus the time of expiration is that the difference in the strength of deformation between the normal liver and the abnormal liver conspicuously varies when the BE/DPS value is calculated when the volume of deformation of the liver is the largest.

The shifts of both BE/DPS values are generally invariant to evaluate the degree of distortion or deformation of a non-rigid object. Rigid movement of the liver by breathing as an affine transform is ignored in the assessment, and only the non-rigid transformation caused by the liver itself is calculated. Although DPS is not rotationally invariant, the rotated element is very small in our datasets because the breathing of patients only makes the liver move up and down. Such properties would make it possible to use BE/DPS values to evaluate the quantitative stiffness of the liver.

Appl. Sci. **2018**, *8*, 437

We assessed that a 12 mm spacing was too small to clearly identify crossing points in the BE/DPS analysis and a 24 mm spacing was too large to have a sufficient number of coordinate samples, especially in small cirrhotic livers. Thus, we chose 16 and 20 mm stripe spacing and sagittal and coronal planes, resulting in four different types of cine-tagging images: 16 mm sagittal, 20 mm sagittal, 16 mm coronal, and 20 mm coronal grids (Figure 1a–d). Comparing the four different types of grids, our preliminary study concluded that the 16 mm sagittal grid with BE features showed the best performance in the diagnosis [19]. For the DPS feature, the performance on these four types of images is shown in Figure 7. The average DPS values in normal and abnormal livers listed in Table 1 indicate that the 16 mm sagittal DPS method also has the best performance, which is identical to the results obtained from the BE method.

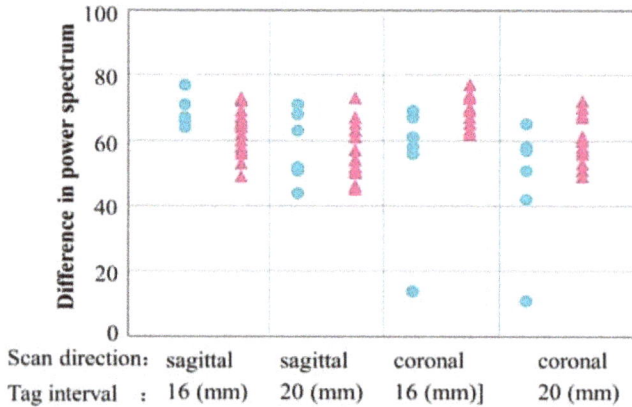

Figure 7. Comparing the DPS values between normal (○) and abnormal cases (▲) in four different types of grids with different scan directions and tag intervals by *t* test, the significance level has the maximum *p* value in 16 mm sagittal grid with $p = 0.05$, which is identical to the results from the BE method.

Table 1. Average values of the difference in the power spectrum (DPS) [1].

Average DPS Values Type of MR Tagging Images	Normal Liver	Abnormal Liver	Difference between Two Groups
16 (mm), sagittal	68.7	62.8	5.9
20 (mm), sagittal	58.2	55.4	2.8
16 (mm), coronal	54.2	69.2	5.0
20 (mm), coronal	47.3	60.7	3.4

[1] MR, magnetic resonance.

The performances based on the bending energy and power spectrum methods shown in Figure 8 are different. Neither of the methods are able to distinguish the abnormal liver from the normal liver. However, the distinction between the normal liver and the abnormal liver becomes much clearer by combining the two methods, as shown in Figure 9. There are many overlap cases in Figure 9a between automatically placing the LMs based on Hough transformation [26] and the automatic DPS value calculation from the original image. Figure 9b is the result of manually placing LMs as the gold standard versus DPS from the segmented liver image. The classification results of Figure 9b obtained by the SOM method in Table 2 demonstrate that 33 cases are successfully classified. One case of the normal liver is falsely classified as abnormal. The follow-up study demonstrates that this false classification may be caused by the subtle breathing action of the healthy patient, which makes the deformation of the liver insufficient.

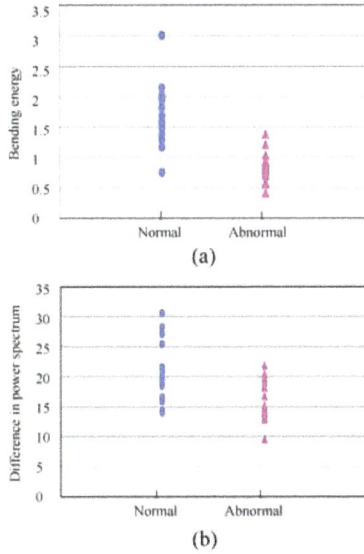

Figure 8. Results of calculated bending energy (**a**) and the differences in power spectra (**b**) for normal (●) and abnormal cases (▲).

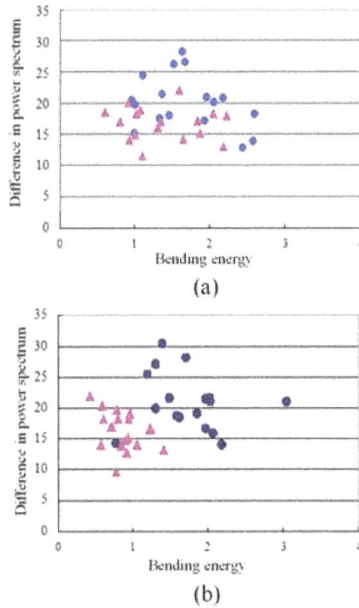

Figure 9. Classification of normal cases (●) from abnormal cases (▲) with two features: bending energy vs. difference in power spectrum by (**a**) automatic placement of landmarks vs. DPS from original image and (**b**) manually placing landmarks vs. DPS from the segmented liver image.

In contrast to the 10+ min required to manually place corresponding landmarks on MR-tagging image pairs, segmentation of the liver region shown in Figure 5 only takes 1–2 min, since the demand for accuracy is not very high, which implies that FFT is faster than time domain processing, as there is no difference in the calculation of BE and DPS values.

Table 2. The classification results for Figure 9b by SOMs (self-organizing maps) with the gold standard.

SOM Gold Standard	Normal Liver	Abnormal Liver
Normal liver	16	0
Abnormal liver	1	17

There are some limitations to our study, and these should be improved upon in future work. First, for the bending energy method, the results change based on the number of LMs used for calculation. Therefore, it is necessary to calculate the bending energy with the same number of the LMs in all cases. Second, this study is based on 2D processing, but liver deformation occurs in three dimensions. Using 3D BE/DPS values may greatly improve the precision of the assessment. Third, this study was conducted as preliminary technical development research, and considerable time and effort were expended to manually define the coordinates and record the values. We have now started to develop an automated algorithm to calculate BE values with cine-tagging MR images, as well as the automatic segmentation of the liver region for calculating the DPS value. Although the results are not yet satisfying, this MR elastography might be more practically incorporated into an MR imaging protocol if the output of the BE/DPS values are fully automated by implementing more intelligent algorithms. Finally, for the abnormal cases, there is no statistical difference between the BE/DPS values with F1/F2 and F3/F4, which is regarded as an important boundary for staging the fibrosis into curable or carcinoma control groups in clinical management. This may be due to either methodological errors in guiding the patients to breath without standard criteria or a low number of experimental datasets. We believe that, with more cases and with a more accurate and efficient liver extraction method, the deformation of tags would have a higher correlation coefficient with the abnormal group. It is possible not only to discriminate fibrotic and cirrhotic livers but also to differentiate individual fibrosis stages by using BE/DPS values or combining them with other effective features [28].

5. Conclusions

This article describes a novel method for measuring the value of non-rigid deformation of the liver in an MR tagging image. In this study, the elasticity of the liver was analyzed by the bending energy and power spectrum on MR tagging images. BE was calculated using a TPS-based method in the spatial domain, and DPS was calculated to quantify the change of tag frequency using the FFT method in the frequency domain. Finally, the abnormal liver was distinguished from the normal liver by using two techniques.

Although the BE and DPS values were not able to distinguish the moderate or advanced hepatic fibrosis from healthy liver or slight hepatic fibrosis successfully, a highly accurate assessment was possible by combining the two methods with the LMs as the gold standard. It is expected that this procedure will be fully automatic with improved accuracy of LM extraction.

This study demonstrated that our proposed method for non-invasively assessing liver fibrosis may be an alternative to traditional liver biopsy without the need for contrast agents or mechanical devices.

Acknowledgments: The authors are grateful to Haruo Watanabe, Masayuki Kanematsu, and members at Fujita lab in Gifu University, for their early efforts and discussions on this research. This work was supported in part by two research support from the National Natural Science Foundation of China (Nos. 81460274 and 81760324), and by JSPS Grant-in-Aid for Scientific Research on Innovative Areas (grant number 26108005), and in part by a research foundation project of the Health and Family planning Commission of Guangxi (No. Z2016762).

Author Contributions: Xiangrong Zhou conceived and designed the experiments; Xuejun Zhang performed the experiments and wrote the paper; Takeshi Hara analyzed the data; Hiroshi Fujita contributed experimental materials.

Conflicts of Interest: The authors declare no conflict of interest.

References

1. El-Serag, H.B.; Mason, A.C. Rising incidence of hepatocellular carcinoma in the United States. *N. Engl. J. Med.* **1999**, *340*, 745–750. [CrossRef] [PubMed]
2. Yatsuhashi, H.; Yano, M. Natural history of chronic hepatitis C. *J. Gastroenterol. Hepatol.* **2000**, *15*, 111–116. [CrossRef]
3. Wynn, T.A. Cellular and molecular mechanisms of fibrosis. *J. Pathol.* **2008**, *214*, 199–210. [CrossRef] [PubMed]
4. Saadeh, S.; Cammell, G.; Carey, W.D.; Younossi, Z.; Barnes, D.; Easley, K. The role of liver biopsy in chronic hepatitis C. *Hepatology* **2001**, *33*, 196–200. [CrossRef] [PubMed]
5. Poynard, T.; Ratziu, V.; Bedossa, P. Appropriateness of liver biopsy. *Can. J. Gastroenterol.* **2000**, *14*, 543–548. [CrossRef] [PubMed]
6. Bravo, A.A.; Sheth, S.G.; Chopra, S. Liver biopsy. *N. Engl. J. Med.* **2001**, *344*, 495–500. [CrossRef] [PubMed]
7. Regev, A.; Berho, M.; Jeffers, L.J.; Milikowski, C.; Molina, E.G.; Pyrsopoulos, N.T.; Feng, Z.Z.; Reddy, K.R.; Schiff, E.R. Sampling error and intraobserver variation in liver biopsy in patients with chronic HCV infection. *Am. J. Gastroenterol.* **2002**, *97*, 2614–2618. [CrossRef] [PubMed]
8. Muthupillai, R.; Lomas, D.J.; Rossman, P.J.; Greenleaf, J.F.; Manduca, A.; Ehman, R.L. Magnetic resonance elastography by direct visualization of propagating acoustic strain waves. *Science* **1995**, *269*, 1854–1857. [CrossRef] [PubMed]
9. Rouviere, O.; Yin, M.; Dresner, M.A.; Rossman, P.J.; Burgart, L.J.; Fidler, J.L.; Ehman, R.L. MR elastography of the liver: Preliminary results. *Radiology* **2006**, *240*, 440–448. [CrossRef] [PubMed]
10. Huwart, L.; Sempoux, C.; Salameh, N.; Jamart, J.; Annet, L.; Sinkus, R.; Peeters, F.; ter Beek, L.C.; Horsmans, Y.; van Beers, B.E. Liver fibrosis: Noninvasive assessment with MR elastography versus aspartate aminotransferase-to-platelet ratio index. *Radiology* **2007**, *245*, 458–466. [CrossRef] [PubMed]
11. Lucidarme, O.; Baleston, F.; Cadi, M.; Bellin, M.F.; Charlotte, F.; Ratziu, V.; Grenier, P.A. Non-invasive detection of liver fibrosis: Is superparamagnetic iron oxide particle-enhanced MR imaging a contributive technique? *Eur. Radiol.* **2002**, *13*, 467–474. [CrossRef] [PubMed]
12. Aguirre, D.A.; Behling, C.A.; Alpert, E.; Hassanein, T.I.; Sirlin, C.B. Liver fibrosis: Noninvasive diagnosis with double contrast material-enhanced MR imaging. *Radiology* **2006**, *239*, 425–437. [CrossRef] [PubMed]
13. Taouli, B.; Tolia, A.J.; Losada, M.; Babb, J.S.; Chan, E.S.; Bannan, M.A.; Tobias, H. Diffusion-weighted MRI for quantification of liver fibrosis: Preliminary experience. *Am. J. Roentgenol.* **2007**, *189*, 799–806. [CrossRef] [PubMed]
14. Friedrich-Rust, M.; Ong, M.F.; Herrmann, E.; Dries, V.; Samaras, P.; Zeuzem, S.; Sarrazin, C. Real-time elastography for noninvasive assessment of liver fibrosis in chronic viral hepatitis. *Am. J. Roentgenol.* **2007**, *188*, 758–764. [CrossRef] [PubMed]
15. Wang, J.; Guo, L.; Shi, X.Y.; Pan, W.Q.; Bai, Y.F.; Ai, H. Real-time elastography with a novel quantitative technology for assessment of liver fibrosis in chronic hepatitis B. *Eur. J. Radiol.* **2012**, *81*, 31–36. [CrossRef] [PubMed]
16. Zhang, X.J.; Li, W.G.; Fujita, H.; Kanematsu, M.; Hara, T.; Zhou, X.R.; Kondo, H.; Hoshi, H. Automatic segmentation of hepatic tissue and 3D volume analysis of cirrhosis in multi-detector row CT scans and MR imaging. *IEICE Trans. Inf. Syst.* **2004**, *87*, 2138–2147.
17. Goshima, S.; Kanematsu, M.; Kobayashi, T.; Furukawa, T.; Zhang, X.; Fujita, H.; Watanabe, H.; Kondo, H.; Moriyama, N.; Bae, K.T. Staging hepatic fibrosis: Computer-aided analysis of hepatic contours on gadolinium ethoxybenzyl diethylenetriaminepentaacetic acid-enhanced hepatocyte-phase magnetic resonance imaging. *Hepatology* **2012**, *55*, 328–329. [CrossRef] [PubMed]
18. Li, W.D.; Zeng, Y.F.; Zhang, X.J.; Huang, Y.; Long, L.L.; Fujita, H. Staging the hepatic fibrosis on CT images: Optimizing the slice thickness and texture features. In Proceedings of the IEEE 2011 International Symposium on Bioelectronics and Bioinformatics, Suzhou, China, 3–5 November 2011; pp. 267–270.

19. Watanabe, H.; Kanematsu, M.; Kitagawa, T.; Suzuki, Y.; Kondo, H.; Goshima, S.; Kajita, K.; Bae, K.T.; Hirose, Y.; Miotani, S.; et al. MR elastography of the liver at 3 T with cine-tagging and bending energy analysis: Preliminary results. *Eur. Radiol.* **2010**, *20*, 2381–2389. [CrossRef] [PubMed]

20. Ohyama, W.; Wakabayashi, T.; Kimura, F.; Tsuruoka, S.; Sekioka, K. Automatic extraction of SPAMM grids in left ventricular myocardium from MR tagging images. In Proceedings of the 2009 International Workshop on Regional Innovation Studies: Biomedical Engineering, Mie, Japan, 8 October 2009; pp. 25–29.

21. Zerhouni, E.A.; Parish, D.M.; Rogers, W.J.; Yang, A.; Shapiro, E.P. Human heart: Tagging with MR imaging—A method for noninvasive assessment of myocardialmotion. *Radiology* **1988**, *169*, 59–63. [CrossRef] [PubMed]

22. Inaba, T.; Kinosada, Y.; Kawasaki, S.; Obata, H.; Tokuda, M. Analysis of left ventricular wall motion using a magnetic resonance tagging technique: Measurement of circumferential elongation of ventricular Wall in Patients with DCM. *Trans. Jpn. Soc. Med. Biol. Eng.* **2003**, *41*, 136–139. (In Japanese)

23. Watanabe, H.; Kanematsu, M.; Kondo, H.; Goshima, S.; Kitagawa, T.; Fujita, H. MR elastography of the liver with cine-tagging and physical bending energy analysis using 3T MRI: Phantom study and preliminary clinical application. In Proceedings of the 94th Scientific Assembly and Annual Meeting of the Radiological Society of North America, Chicago, IL, USA, 30 November–5 December 2008; p. 828.

24. Axel, L.; Dougherty, L. MR imaging of motion with spatial modulation of magnetization. *Radiology* **1989**, *171*, 841–845. [CrossRef] [PubMed]

25. Bookstein, F.L. Principal warps: Thin-plate splines and the decomposition of deformations. *IEEE Trans. Pattern Anal. Mach. Intell.* **1989**, *11*, 567–585.

26. Miotani, S.; Zhou, X.G.; Kitagawa, T.; Hara, T.; Fujita, H.; Yokoyama, R.; Watanae, H.; Kanematsu, M.; Hoshi, H. *Initial Examination of Automatic Calculation Method of Non-Rigid Deformity of the Liver in MR Tagging Images*; IEICE Technical Report; IEICE: Minato-ku, Tokyo, 2009; Volume 109, pp. 213–218. (In Japanese)

27. Hosseini, H.S.; Safabakhsh, R. TASOM: A New Time Adaptive Self-Organizing Map. *IEEE Trans. Syst. Man Cybern.* **2003**, *33*, 271–282. [CrossRef] [PubMed]

28. Zhang, X.J.; Goshima, S.; Zhou, X.G.; Hara, T.; Kanematsu, M.; Fujita, H.; Furukawa, T. Quantitative staging the hepatic Fibrosis: Computer-aided diagnosis by shape, texture, volume, and elasticity analysis. In Proceedings of the Radiological Society of North America 2011 Scientific Assembly and Annual Meeting, Chicago, IL, USA, 26 November–2 December 2011.

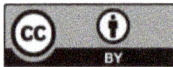

© 2018 by the authors. Licensee MDPI, Basel, Switzerland. This article is an open access article distributed under the terms and conditions of the Creative Commons Attribution (CC BY) license (http://creativecommons.org/licenses/by/4.0/).

applied
sciences

MDPI

Article

Ultrasound-Based Liver Stiffness Surveillance in Patients Treated for Chronic Hepatitis B or C

Sheng-Hung Chen [1,2,3] and **Cheng-Yuan Peng** [2,3,*]

1   Graduate Institute of Clinical Medical Science, School of Medicine, China Medical University,
    Taichung 40447, Taiwan; d14675@mail.cmuh.org.tw
2   School of Medicine, China Medical University, Taichung 40402, Taiwan
3   Division of Hepatogastroenterology, Department of Internal Medicine, China Medical University Hospital,
    Taichung 40447, Taiwan
*   Correspondence: cypeng@mail.cmuh.org.tw; Tel.: +886-4-2205-2121 (ext. 2260); Fax: +886-4-2207-1600

Received: 9 March 2018; Accepted: 30 March 2018; Published: 17 April 2018

Abstract: Evolving modes of ultrasound-based elastography have achieved promising validity and reliability for evaluating liver fibrosis. Liver stiffness (LS) is a valuable biomarker for modeling liver disease progression and regression on a continuous noncategorical scale as changes in LS per year or for determining the LS progression or regression rate for refining LS measurement (LSM)-based prognostics. The paradigm of LSMs has altered the focus from liver fibrosis staging alone to comprehensive liver-relevant risk estimations. However, diverse ranges of cohort characteristics, disease types, surveillance protocols and timeframes, necroinflammatory resolutions or biochemical responses (BRs), factors explaining the magnitude or kinetics in LS change, virologic responses (VRs), fibrosis reversals (FRs), and noninvasive surveillance results have rarely been reviewed collectively. Elastography-based LS surveillance alone conveys chronological and valuable patient information and assists in characterizing worldwide patient cohorts under antiviral treatment by delineating the concurrent time elapsed, VR, BR, and FR. In groups with uniform VRs to direct-acting antivirals for chronic hepatitis C and nucleoside and nucleotide analogs for chronic hepatitis B, decline in LS can be explained using concurrent BR from 24 weeks to 3 years, followed by FR and the time elapsed.

Keywords: elastography; liver stiffness; chronic hepatitis B; chronic hepatitis C; liver fibrosis; cirrhosis

1. Introduction

Chronic hepatitis (CH) B and C treatment is a major global healthcare challenge. Antiviral treatment can alter natural history and reduce risks of cirrhosis, hepatic decompensation, and hepatocellular carcinoma [1,2]. Antiviral therapy in patients with CHB with decompensated cirrhosis improves hepatic reserve and reduces mortality [2,3]. With the advent of direct-acting antivirals (DAAs) for CHC, recent studies have demonstrated that DAA therapy can improve hepatic reserve and delay progression in patients with CHC with decompensated cirrhosis [4]. Furthermore, most patients with CHB or CHC—even those without a treatment response—benefit from antiviral treatment, evidenced by a marked early resolution in hepatic necroinflammation [5,6] and a fibrosis reversal over time [7,8].

However, a virologic response to CHB or CHC treatment does not ensure zero risk of liver-related adverse endpoints after virologic response [9–11]. Therefore, both on-treatment and off-treatment parameters over time should be investigated to further gain insight into the natural history and treatment-modified disease course of chronic viral hepatitis [10–12].

Elastography noninvasively quantifies tissue elasticity and stiffness. By using external or internal impulses, elastographic techniques determine tissue stiffness by calculating tissue strains or shear wave velocities [13]. Currently, in noninvasive liver fibrosis evaluation in either a clinical or research setting [14], baseline liver stiffness is a well-established and promising noninvasive biomarker for assessing pretreatment fibrosis in patients with chronic liver diseases [15] and for predicting liver-related events [16]. The evolving modes of ultrasound-based elastography possess promising and comparable validity and reliability for evaluating fibrosis [17,18], despite the limitations, ranging from poor acoustic windows to the motion effects related to measurement variability [19].

Recent studies have further revealed that liver stiffness measurement is a promising solution to modeling liver disease progression and regression on a continuous noncategorical scale as changes in liver stiffness per year or liver stiffness progression or regression rate to refine liver stiffness measurement-based prognostics [7,20–23]. Regarding the heterogeneous surveillance intervals in reports using liver stiffness measurements, the durations were significantly shorter either during treatment or between the end of treatment (EOT) and follow-up in patients with CHB and CHC than those reported in histological studies with follow-up periods of up to 10 years [24,25]. Studies applying paired liver biopsies (pre- and post-antiviral treatment) have reported rates of cirrhosis reversal of up to 74% of patients with CHB and 18–64% of patients with CHC with cirrhosis over long-term intervals of up to 5 and 10 years, respectively [9,24–26]. Nonetheless, the paradigms of liver stiffness measurements have shifted focus from the outdated cross-sectional liver fibrosis staging alone to comprehensive liver-relevant risk estimation [27]. However, diverse ranges of cohort characteristics, disease types, surveillance protocols and timeframes, and necroinflammatory resolution or biochemical responses, factors explaining the magnitude or kinetics in liver stiffness change, virologic responses, fibrosis reversals, and noninvasive surveillance results have rarely been reviewed collectively [28].

In this study, we searched and reviewed representative reports on liver stiffness surveillance with no less than two surveillance visits in PubMed, Medline, and Cochrane Library databases for papers published between January 2010 and January 2018. Articles not written in English were excluded.

2. CHC

Among liver fibrosis surveillance reports of patients with CHC, comparisons were made in terms of the therapy (including the untreated group), kinetics of liver stiffness, time elapsed, virologic response, and biochemical response (Table 1).

A study [29] reported the kinetics and correlates of liver stiffness over an elapsed time on 126 patients with CHC who received pegIFN-based therapy. At the EOT, 48 weeks after the EOT, and 96 weeks after the EOT, liver stiffness declined significantly from the baseline in the group with sustained virologic response (SVR; $n = 57$; -16.2%, -32.2%, and -43.5% change, respectively) compared with the non-SVR group ($n = 69$; -7.2%, -2.1%, and $+17.3\%$ change, respectively; $p = 0.0127$, $p < 0.0001$, and $p < 0.0001$, respectively). After further stratification by biochemical responses, at the EOT, 48 weeks after the EOT, and 96 weeks after the EOT, liver stiffness still declined significantly in patients with a biochemical response ($n = 16$; -17.9%, -30.0%, and -27.1%, respectively) compared with the group without a biochemical response ($n = 53$; -4.1%, $+6.4\%$, and $+30.6\%$, respectively; $p = 0.0270$, $p < 0.0001$, and $p < 0.0001$, respectively) among patients without SVR. Therefore, both virologic response and biochemical response influenced the decline in liver stiffness.

In another study including 180 patients [30], liver stiffness declined significantly from the baseline in the SVR ($n = 93$) and relapse ($n = 28$) groups, but not in the nonresponder ($n = 24$) or untreated ($n = 35$) group. Correlation among the declines in liver stiffness were further estimated through univariate and multiple regressions in the group with relatively high pretreatment liver stiffness values (deduced as METAVIR F3 or F4 stages, $n = 67$). This indicated that the beneficial effects of pegIFN-based therapy on the decline in liver stiffness were independently associated with milder fibrosis stage (also indicated by a lower hyaluronic acid level), more severe inflammatory activity (indicated by a higher alanine aminotransferase (ALT) level) at the baseline, virologic response, and a longer pegIFN therapy course. The reason for this result is that liver stiffness typically reflects the degrees of both fibrosis and necroinflammation and that pretreatment fibrosis is inversely correlated with treatment response.

SVR is approximately equivalent to the cessation of viral replication, necroinflammation, and fibrosis progression [31]. Patients with long-term virus-eradicated status after SVR develop fewer adverse outcomes, such as cirrhosis, decompensation, and hepatocellular carcinoma, than those without SVR do. In general, post-treatment SVR status outweighed baseline hepatitis C virus (HCV) RNA in the studies to correlate with significant declines in liver stiffness. Apart from studies in which the cohorts were not stratified [32–36], non-SVR generally accounted for nonsignificant declines in liver stiffness. However, those who experienced a relapse in the non-SVR group still could exhibit significant declines in liver stiffness [30,37,38]. In the untreated groups recruited in various studies [29,30,37], nonsignificant declines in liver stiffness were observed throughout the timeframes. However, SVR does not necessarily terminate the progression of disease course, particularly in patients with advanced cirrhosis at the baseline [4]. In a cohort of patients (*n* = 226) with HCV-related cirrhosis and clinically significant portal hypertension (CSPH) receiving DAA therapy, hepatic vein pressure gradient decreased by 10% in 62% of patients but CSPH persisted in 78% of patients despite achieving SVR. One third of patients with a reduction in liver stiffness measurement to below 13.6 kPa (cutoff for ruling out CSPH at the baseline) after SVR still had CSPH, indicating the suboptimal discriminative capacity of liver stiffness measurement for patients with CSPH after an SVR [22].

In addition to stratification by the SVR status, baseline liver stiffness values outweighed SVRs in the various regression analyses adopting various baseline and chronological host and viral covariates to explain the declines in liver stiffness [37–40] (Table 1). Declines in liver stiffness tended to be greater in patients with higher baseline liver stiffness values, reflecting the effects of biochemical response on liver stiffness over time [29]. Moreover, the heterogeneity of liver stiffness declines in the group without an SVR (i.e., in several studies, those who relapsed still could achieve a significant reduction in liver stiffness) [30,37,38] also contributed to the nonsignificant effect of SVR status on the declines in liver stiffness over time. In a recent study [38], approximately 80% of patients experienced a decline in paired liver stiffness values from the baseline to the SVR visit in the stratified subgroups. The overall percentages of patients who exhibited any decline in liver stiffness did not differ significantly among the SVR (80.8%, 177/219), relapse (77.8%, 21/27), and nonresponse (80.0%, 8/10) groups. Similarly, in a previous study [41], 250 (76.2%) out of 328 patients who received DAA-based therapy and paired liver stiffness measurements exhibited an improvement in liver stiffness from the baseline to the SVR visit 12 weeks after treatment.

After adjustment for other baseline covariates through regression analyses, several individual non-pooling studies [30,35,37] identified baseline hepatic necroinflammation or a necroinflammatory decline over time from the study entry date as being significantly correlated with a decline in liver stiffness. Biochemical responses were also revealed to be in parallel with the liver stiffness decline over time [38]. However, only one study has analyzed the two-phased liver stiffness declines or the rapid-to-slow rates of liver stiffness kinetics (typically declines) through liver stiffness surveillance at shorter time intervals by including patients with CHB [7]. Among the noninvasive liver fibrosis evaluation approaches or indices, elastography-based liver stiffness measurements in particular were affected at an early stage by hepatic necroinflammatory activity [32]. The activity typically remained relatively stable over the later phase. After ALT normalization, liver stiffness continued to decline gradually, reflecting the ongoing occurrence of fibrosis reversal over time [7,8]. Therefore, lower cutoff values than those acquired at the treatment baseline have been recommended for surveillance by dichotomizing the fibrosis stages in patients with CHC using elastography on and off treatments [32,34,42]. Furthermore, a large-scale study is required to validate these proposed cutoff values for the prediction of fibrosis stage in treatment-experienced patients. Moreover, experiences in both clinical and research settings have revealed concordances and discordances between different fibrosis evaluation measures [43]. However, a combination of evaluation measures may enhance diagnostic performance [43,44].

Despite the lack of a critical evaluation of the potential for publication bias and quality and pooling of the original data for overall estimations among the reviewed contributions, the current study provides valuable perspectives regarding liver stiffness surveillance.

In addition to virologic response and biochemical response, surges in the trajectories of liver stiffness values over time may provide a warning for conditions such as hyperbilirubinemia or excessive necroinflammatory flare-ups, particularly during DAA therapy for CHC, excessive alcohol consumption, exposure to hepatotoxins, viral reactivations, superinfections, or relapses. Among patients that ordinarily experience declining liver stiffness values over time, any marked increase in liver stiffness may prompt medical professionals to implement further differential diagnoses for the examinee, potentially requiring further medical attention at any time point during surveillance. The rates of decline (or progression) in liver stiffness may be compared between the pegIFN- and DAA-based groups. Moreover, liver stiffness surveillance may assist in stratifying the patients with CHC according to early and late rates of decline (or progression) in liver stiffness to implement estimates through time-dependent approaches [45] or decision-tree algorithms [46] for future liver-related endpoints.

Table 1. Published studies on liver stiffness surveillance in patients with chronic hepatitis C.

Study/Year	Size	Therapy (Based)	Off-Treatment Timeframes	Groups with Nonsignificant LS Declines	Groups with Significant [a] LS Declines	LS-Decline Correlates [b]	SVR-Status Correlates [b]
Ogawa 2009 [29]	145	PegIFN	EOT-wk48–wk96	NSVR with no BR/untreated	SVR/NSVR with BR	NA	NA
Arima 2010 [30]	180	IFN\PegIFN	EOT-wk48–wk96	Nonresponders/untreated	SVR/relapsers	Milder fibrosis stages, lower hyaluronic acid levels, longer pegIFN treatment, SVR, higher ALT levels in the group with higher baseline LS values (deduced F3, F4)	NA
Wang 2010 [39]	144	IFN\pegIFN	EOT-y5	NSVR	SVR	Rapid LS declines: higher baseline LS; slow LS declines: advanced pretreatment fibrosis stages/higher BMI/longer time remission	NA
Hézode 2011 [47]	91	PegIFN	EOT-wk24	NSVR	SVR	SVR	NA
Martinez 2012 [35]	515	PegIFN	EOT-wk72	Non-responders/untreated	SVR/relapsers	Higher baseline LS/ALT levels/antiviral therapy/non-1 genotypes	NA
Stasi 2013 [48]	49	PegIFN	EOT-wk144	NSVR	SVR	SVR	NA
Salmon 2015 [40]	98 [c]	PegIFN\DAA	EOT-y3	NSVR	SVR	SVR/higher baseline LS/lower AST	NA
Moser 2016 [32]	53	DAA	On-treatment follow-up alone (1–6 wk from baseline)	No stratified groups	No stratified groups	NA	NA
Bachofner 2017 [33]	392	DAA	EOT-wk72	No stratified groups	No stratified groups	NA	NA
Chan 2017 [35]	70	DAA	EOT-wk48	No stratified groups	No stratified groups	Higher baseline ALT level/HCV genotype 1	NA
Elsharkawy 2017 [41]	337	DAA	EOT-wk12	Relapsers	SVR	Correlated with non improvement in LS: relapsers/lower baseline LS	NA
Tada 2017 [46]	210	DAA	EOT-wk24	No stratified groups	No stratified groups	NA	NA
Tachi 2018 [44]	176	PegIFN\DAA	EOT-wk24	No stratified groups	No stratified groups	Higher baseline necroinflammatory activity for LS declines till EOT/significant baseline fibrosis stages for LS declines till 24 wk after EOT	NA
Łucejko 2018 [49]	34	DAA	EOT-wk24–wk96	No stratified groups	No stratified groups	Advanced baseline fibrosis stages/higher ALT/lower HCVcAg	NA
Chen 2018 [38]	256	PegIFN\DAA	EOT-wk24	Non-responders	SVR/relapsers	Higher baseline LS/lower BMI	Lower baseline LS/lower BMI/IL 28B polymorphisms/RVR

ALT, alanine aminotransferase; AST, aspartate aminotransferase; BMI, body mass index; BR, biochemical response; DAA, direct-acting antiviral; EOT, end of treatment; HCV, hepatitis C virus; HCVcAg, hepatitis C virus core antigen; LS, liver stiffness; NA, not available; NSVR, non-sustained virologic response; pegIFN, pegylated interferon; SVR, sustained virologic response; wk, week; y, year; LS decline, defined as the value equal to the baseline minus the follow-up; [a] the time elapsed varied among studies that were fixed or time-dependent; [b] the correlates with LS-decline and SVR: acquired through multiple regression analysis; [c] human immunodeficiency virus/HCV-coinfected.

3. CHB

Compared with CHC, the baseline liver stiffness values remained the most crucial of all factors to explain the liver stiffness improvement over follow-up periods (Table 2). Except in the study [50], employing the absolute value of follow-up liver stiffness (<7.2 kPa on FibroScan) as the outcome, participants with lower baseline liver stiffness were more likely to achieve favorable outcome than those with higher liver stiffness values.

Table 2. Published studies on liver stiffness surveillance in patients with chronic hepatitis B.

Study/Year	Size	Follow-Up Timeframes	Baseline Pathology	Multiple Biopsies	LS-Decline Correlates
Ogawa 2011 [52]	45	Baseline–yearly–y5/y3–y5	Yes	No	NA
Fung 2011 [51]	426	Baseline–y3	No	No	Subsequent ALT normalization in the treated/persistently normal ALT in the untreated groups
Kim 2014 [53]	83	411.5 ± 149.5 days	No	No	NA
Liang 2017 [7]	534	Baseline–wk24–wk102	Yes	Yes	[a] Higher changes of Ishak stage
Li 2017 [54]	334	24wk	No	No	Higher baseline AST/lower ALT/higher α-fetoprotein/higher LS/longer course of antiviral therapy
Chon 2017 [50]	120	Baseline–yearly–y5	Yes	No	Lower baseline LS values (<12.0 kPa)
Wu 2017 [8]	71	Baseline–wk26–wk53–wk78–wk104	Yes	Yes	Higher baseline LS
Rinaldi 2018 [55]	189	Baseline–wk24	No	No	Higher baseline LS
Li 2018 [56]	104	Baseline–y3	Yes	No	NA

LS, liver stiffness; wk, week; y, year; LS decline, defined as the value equal to the baseline minus the follow-up; NA, not available; [a] for the group with paired liver biopsies.

In addition, time elapsed and biochemical response typically superseded the baseline hepatitis B virus DNA, viral genotypes, serology, and several host factors, in their correlation with a decline in liver stiffness [7]. The liver stiffness surveillance of the CHB cohort was not grouped by virologic response because of the uniform virologic response to antiviral treatment with nucleoside or nucleotide analogs.

Regarding biochemical response, either absolute ALT values or declines in ALT levels rarely showed direct significance after regression analyses. The correlations between necroinflammatory degrees and liver stiffness declines were mostly demonstrated through groups stratified by changes in ALT levels [51] and by the results that changes in ALT levels were parallel with declines in liver stiffness [7].

Few studies have implemented paired liver biopsies to assess the fibrosis reversal. In a study [7], fibrosis reversal was observed in 98 (59.8%) of 164 patients; these 164 (30.7%) patients were selected from 534 study participants receiving adequate paired liver biopsies at the baseline and week 104 over the course of CHB treatment. Of the 98 patients with fibrosis reversal, 63 (64.3%), 22 (22.4%), 10 (10.2%), and 3 (3.1%) exhibited 1-, 2-, 3-, and 4-point declines in Ishak fibrosis stages, respectively. After adjustment for changes in ALT and Knodell scores, changes in Ishak fibrosis stage were independently associated with declines in liver stiffness measurement of greater than 30% from the baseline to week 104 (odds ratio, 1.466; 95% confidence interval, 1.079–1.992; $p = 0.014$).

In another study [8], 27 patients received paired liver biopsies. Among the 14 patients with a significant decline in liver stiffness of ≥15% from the baseline to week 78, up to 12 (85.7%) experienced fibrosis reversal (decline in METAVIR fibrosis ≥ 1 stage). Among the 13 patients with static liver stiffness values, 10 (76.9%) had stable fibrosis stages on histology, whereas 3 (23.1%) had fibrosis reversal. The Spearman's rank correlation analysis revealed significant correlations between declines in liver stiffness and changes in histological fibrosis stages ($r = 0.63$, $p < 0.001$).

Appl. Sci. **2018**, *8*, 626

Therefore, biochemical response, followed by fibrosis reversal and time elapsed, but not the virologic response, aided in understanding of the liver stiffness kinetics in the CHB cohort under surveillance.

In conclusion, liver stiffness could be a promising and significant biomarker in evaluating CHC or CHB across on- and off-treatment timeframes [44,57]. Elastography-based liver-stiffness surveillance alone conveys chronological and informative patient information. In addition, it facilitates the characterization of patient cohorts undergoing antiviral treatment worldwide by collaboratively delineating the time elapsed, virologic response, biochemical response, and fibrosis reversal. In groups with uniform virologic responses to DAAs for CHC and nucleoside and nucleotide analogs for CHB, declines in liver stiffness can be explained by the early concurrent biochemical response over time (from 24 weeks to 3 years), followed by fibrosis reversal and time elapsed. Future studies should quantify the concurrent true liver collagen content and define the fibrosis stage to help specify the kinetics and validate the cutoff values of liver stiffness when dichotomizing fibrosis stages over time.

Acknowledgments: This review was supported in part by a grant (MOST 104-2314-B-039-014) from the Ministry of Science and Technology, Taiwan. This manuscript was edited by Wallace Academic Editing.

Author Contributions: Sheng-Hung Chen and Cheng-Yuan Peng performed the reviews; Sheng-Hung Chen and Cheng-Yuan Peng wrote the paper.

Conflicts of Interest: The authors declare no conflicts of interest.

References

1. Van der Meer, A.J.; Wedemeyer, H.; Feld, J.J.; Hansen, B.E.; Manns, M.P.; Zeuzem, S.; Janssen, H.L. Is there sufficient evidence to recommend antiviral therapy in hepatitis C? *J. Hepatol.* **2014**, *60*, 191–196. [CrossRef] [PubMed]
2. Lok, A.S.; McMahon, B.J.; Brown, R.S., Jr.; Wong, J.B.; Ahmed, A.T.; Farah, W.; Almasri, J.; Alahdab, F.; Benkhadra, K.; Mouchli, M.A.; et al. Antiviral therapy for chronic hepatitis B viral infection in adults: A systematic review and meta-analysis. *Hepatology* **2016**, *63*, 284–306. [CrossRef] [PubMed]
3. Peng, C.Y.; Chien, R.N.; Liaw, Y.F. Hepatitis B virus-related decompensated liver cirrhosis: Benefits of antiviral therapy. *J. Hepatol.* **2012**, *57*, 442–450. [CrossRef] [PubMed]
4. Curry, M.P. Direct acting antivirals for decompensated cirrhosis. Efficacy and safety are now established. *J. Hepatol.* **2016**, *64*, 1206–1207. [CrossRef] [PubMed]
5. Liang, X.E.; Chen, Y.P.; Zhang, Q.; Dai, L.; Zhu, Y.F.; Hou, J.L. Dynamic evaluation of liver stiffness measurement to improve diagnostic accuracy of liver cirrhosis in patients with chronic hepatitis B acute exacerbation. *J. Viral Hepat.* **2011**, *18*, 884–891. [CrossRef] [PubMed]
6. Tada, T.; Kumada, T.; Toyoda, H.; Sone, Y.; Takeshima, K.; Ogawa, S.; Goto, T.; Wakahata, A.; Nakashima, M.; Nakamuta, M.; et al. Viral eradication reduces both LS and steatosis in patients with chronic hepatitis C virus infection who received direct-acting anti-viral therapy. *Aliment. Pharmacol. Ther.* **2018**, *47*, 1012–1022. [CrossRef] [PubMed]
7. Liang, X.; Xie, Q.; Tan, D.; Ning, Q.; Niu, J.; Bai, X.; Chen, S.; Cheng, J.; Yu, Y.; Wang, H.; et al. Interpretation of liver stiffness measurement-based approach for the monitoring of hepatitis B patients with antiviral therapy: A 2-year prospective study. *J. Viral Hepat.* **2017**, *25*, 296–305. [CrossRef] [PubMed]
8. Wu, S.D.; Ding, H.; Liu, L.L.; Zhuang, Y.; Liu, Y.; Cheng, L.S.; Wang, S.Q.; Tseng, Y.J.; Wang, J.Y.; Jiang, W. Longitudinal monitoring of liver stiffness by acoustic radiation force impulse imaging in patients with chronic hepatitis B receiving entecavir. *Clin. Res. Hepatol. Gastroenterol.* **2017**. [CrossRef] [PubMed]
9. Poynard, T.; Moussalli, J.; Munteanu, M.; Thabut, D.; Lebray, P.; Rudler, M.; Ngo, Y.; Thibault, V.; Mkada, H.; Charlotte, F.; Bismut, F.; Deckmyn, O.; et al. Slow regression of liver fibrosis presumed by repeated biomarkers after virological cure in patients with chronic hepatitis C. *J. Hepatol.* **2013**, *59*, 675–683. [CrossRef] [PubMed]
10. Lee, M.H.; Huang, C.F.; Lai, H.C.; Lin, C.Y.; Dai, C.Y.; Liu, C.J.; Wang, J.H.; Huang, J.F.; Su, W.P.; Yang, H.C.; et al. Clinical efficacy and post-treatment seromarkers associated with the risk of hepatocellular carcinoma among chronic hepatitis C patients. *Sci. Rep.* **2017**, *7*, 3718. [CrossRef] [PubMed]

11. Chen, C.H.; Lee, C.M.; Lai, H.C.; Hu, T.H.; Su, W.P.; Lu, S.N.; Lin, C.H.; Hung, C.H.; Wang, J.H.; Lee, M.H.; et al. Prediction model of hepatocellular carcinoma risk in Asian patients with chronic hepatitis B treated with entecavir. *Oncotarget* **2017**, *8*, 92431–92441. [CrossRef] [PubMed]

12. Yu, M.L.; Huang, C.F.; Yeh, M.L.; Tsai, P.C.; Huang, C.I.; Hsieh, M.H.; Hsieh, M.Y.; Lin, Z.Y.; Chen, S.C.; Huang, J.F.; et al. Time-degenerative factors and the risk of hepatocellular carcinoma after antiviral therapy among hepatitis C virus patients: A model for prioritization of treatment. *Clin. Cancer Res.* **2017**, *23*, 1690–1697. [CrossRef] [PubMed]

13. Sigrist, R.M.S.; Liau, J.; Kaffas, A.E.; Chammas, M.C.; Willmann, J.K. Ultrasound elastography: Review of techniques and clinical applications. *Theranostics* **2017**, *7*, 1303–1329. [CrossRef] [PubMed]

14. Trivedi, H.D.; Lin, S.C.; Lau, D.T.Y. Noninvasive assessment of fibrosis regression in hepatitis C virus sustained virologic responders. *Gastroenterol. Hepatol.* **2017**, *13*, 587–595.

15. Summers, J.A.; Radhakrishnan, M.; Morris, E.; Chalkidou, A.; Rua, T.; Patel, A.; McMillan, V.; Douiri, A.; Wang, Y.; Ayis, S.; Higgins, J.; et al. Virtual Touch™ Quantification to diagnose and monitor liver fibrosis in hepatitis B and hepatitis C: A NICE medical technology guidance. *Appl. Health Econ. Health Policy* **2017**, *15*, 139–154. [CrossRef] [PubMed]

16. Lee, H.W.; Yoo, E.J.; Kim, B.K.; Kim, S.U.; Park, J.Y.; Kim, D.Y.; Ahn, S.H.; Han, K.H. Prediction of development of liver-related events by transient elastography in hepatitis B patients with complete virological response on antiviral therapy. *Am. J. Gastroenterol.* **2014**, *109*, 1241–1249. [CrossRef] [PubMed]

17. Ferraioli, G.; Filice, C.; Castera, L.; Choi, B.I.; Sporea, I.; Wilson, S.R.; Cosgrove, D.; Dietrich, C.F.; Amy, D.; Bamber, J.C.; et al. WFUMB guidelines and recommendations for clinical use of ultrasound elastography: Part 3: Liver. *Ultrasound Med. Biol.* **2015**, *41*, 1161–1179. [CrossRef] [PubMed]

18. Kennedy, P.; Wagner, M.; Castéra, L.; Hong, C.W.; Johnson, C.L.; Sirlin, C.B.; Taouli, B. Quantitative elastography methods in liver disease: Current evidence and future directions. *Radiology* **2018**, *286*, 738–763. [CrossRef] [PubMed]

19. Shin, H.J.; Kim, M.J.; Yoon, C.S.; Lee, K.; Lee, K.S.; Park, J.C.; Lee, M.J.; Yoon, H. Motion effects on the measurement of stiffness on ultrasound shear wave elastography: A moving liver fibrosis phantom study. *Med. Ultrasongr.* **2018**, *1*, 14–20. [CrossRef] [PubMed]

20. Christiansen, K.M.; Mössner, B.K.; Hansen, J.F.; Jarnbjer, E.F.; Pedersen, C.; Christensen, P.B. Liver stiffness measurement among patients with chronic hepatitis B and C: Results from a 5-year prospective study. *PLoS ONE* **2014**, *9*, e111912. [CrossRef] [PubMed]

21. Erman, A.; Sathya, A.; Nam, A.; Bielecki, J.M.; Feld, J.J.; Thein, H.H.; Wong, W.W.L.; Grootendorst, P.; Krahn, M.D. Estimating chronic hepatitis C prognosis using transient elastography-based liver stiffness: A systematic review and meta-analysis. *J. Viral. Hepat.* **2017**. [CrossRef] [PubMed]

22. Lens, S.; Alvarado-Tapias, E.; Mariño, Z.; Londoño, M.C.; LLop, E.; Martinez, J.; Fortea, J.I.; Ibañez, L.; Ariza, X.; Baiges, A.; et al. Effects of all-oral anti-viral therapy on HVPG and systemic hemodynamics in patients with hepatitis C virus-associated cirrhosis. *Gastroenterology* **2017**, *153*, 1273–1283. [CrossRef] [PubMed]

23. Kamarajah, S.K.; Chan, W.K.; Nik Mustapha, N.R.; Mahadeva, S. Repeated liver stiffness measurement compared with paired liver biopsy in patients with non-alcoholic fatty liver disease. *Hepatol. Int.* **2018**, *12*, 44–55. [CrossRef] [PubMed]

24. Gonzalez, H.C.; Duarte-Rojo, A. Virologic cure of hepatitis C: Impact on hepatic fibrosis and patient outcomes. *Curr. Gastroenterol. Rep.* **2016**, *18*, 32. [CrossRef] [PubMed]

25. Shiratori, Y.; Imazeki, F.; Moriyama, M.; Yano, M.; Arakawa, Y.; Yokosuka, O.; Kuroki, T.; Nishiguchi, S.; Sata, M.; Yamada, G.; et al. Histologic improvement of fibrosis in patients with hepatitis C who have sustained response to interferon therapy. *Ann. Intern. Med.* **2000**, *132*, 517–524. [CrossRef] [PubMed]

26. Marcellin, P.; Gane, E.; Buti, M.; Afdhal, N.; Sievert, W.; Jacobson, I.M.; Washington, M.K.; Germanidis, G.; Flaherty, J.F.; Aguilar Schall, R.; et al. Regression of cirrhosis during treatment with tenofovir disoproxil fumarate for chronic hepatitis B: A 5-year open-label follow-up study. *Lancet* **2013**, *381*, 468–475. [CrossRef]

27. Tapper, E.B.; Afdhal, N.H. Chapter 8 Noninvasive assessment of disease progression. In *Zakim and Boyer's Hepatology*, 7th ed.; Boyer, T.D., Sanyal, A.J., Terrault, N.A., Lindor, K.D., Eds.; Elsevier: Amsterdam, The Netherlands, 2017; pp. 117–126, ISBN 9780323446570, 9780323446563.

28. Singh, S.; Facciorusso, A.; Loomba, R.; Falck-Ytter, Y.T. Magnitude and kinetics of decrease in liver stiffness after anti-viral therapy in patients with chronic hepatitis C: A systematic review and meta-analysis. *Clin. Gastroenterol. Hepatol.* **2018**, *16*, 27–38. [CrossRef] [PubMed]

29. Ogawa, E.; Furusyo, N.; Toyoda, K.; Takeoka, H.; Maeda, S.; Hayashi, J. The longitudinal quantitative assessment by transient elastography of chronic hepatitis C patients treated with pegylated interferon alpha-2b and ribavirin. *Antivir. Res.* **2009**, *83*, 127–134. [CrossRef] [PubMed]

30. Arima, Y.; Kawabe, N.; Hashimoto, S.; Harata, M.; Nitta, Y.; Murao, M.; Nakano, T.; Shimazaki, H.; Kobayashi, K.; Ichino, N.; et al. Reduction of liver stiffness by interferon treatment in the patients with chronic hepatitis C. *Hepatol. Res.* **2010**, *40*, 383–392. [CrossRef] [PubMed]

31. Mauro, E.; Crespo, G.; Montironi, C.; Londoño, M.C.; Díaz, A.; Forns, X.; Navasa, M. Viral eradication and fibrosis resolution in post liver transplant cholestatic hepatitis C. *Liver Transpl.* **2018**. [CrossRef] [PubMed]

32. Moser, S.; Gutic, E.; Schleicher, M.; Gschwantler, M. Early decrease of liver stiffness after initiation of antiviral therapy in patients with chronic hepatitis C. *Dig. Liver Dis.* **2016**, *48*, 970–971. [CrossRef] [PubMed]

33. Bachofner, J.A.; Valli, P.V.; Kröger, A.; Bergamin, I.; Künzler, P.; Baserga, A.; Braun, D.; Seifert, B.; Moncsek, A.; Fehr, J.; et al. Direct antiviral agent treatment of chronic hepatitis C results in rapid regression of transient elastography and fibrosis markers fibrosis-4 score and aspartate aminotransferase-platelet ratio index. *Liver Int.* **2017**, *37*, 369–376. [CrossRef] [PubMed]

34. Tachi, Y.; Hirai, T.; Kojima, Y.; Ishizu, Y.; Honda, T.; Kuzuya, T.; Hayashi, K.; Ishigami, M.; Goto, H. Liver stiffness reduction correlates with histological characteristics of hepatitis C patients with sustained virological response. *Liver Int.* **2018**, *38*, 59–67.

35. Chan, J.; Gogela, N.; Zheng, H.; Lammert, S.; Ajayi, T.; Fricker, Z.; Kim, A.Y.; Robbins, G.K.; Chung, R.T. Direct-acting antiviral therapy for chronic HCV infection results in liver stiffness regression over 12 months post-treatment. *Dig. Dis. Sci.* **2018**, *63*, 486–492. [CrossRef] [PubMed]

36. Tada, T.; Kumada, T.; Toyoda, H.; Mizuno, K.; Sone, Y.; Kataoka, S.; Hashinokuchi, S. Improvement of liver stiffness in patients with hepatitis C virus infection who received direct-acting antiviral therapy and achieved sustained virological response. *J. Gastroenterol. Hepatol.* **2017**, *32*, 1982–1988. [CrossRef] [PubMed]

37. Martinez, S.M.; Foucher, J.; Combis, J.M.; Métivier, S.; Brunetto, M.; Capron, D.; Bourlière, M.; Bronowicki, J.P.; Dao, T.; Maynard-Muet, M.; et al. Longitudinal liver stiffness assessment in patients with chronic hepatitis C undergoing antiviral therapy. *PLoS ONE* **2012**, *7*, e47715. [CrossRef] [PubMed]

38. Chen, S.H.; Lai, H.C.; Chiang, I.P.; Su, W.P.; Lin, C.H.; Kao, J.T.; Chuang, P.H.; Hsu, W.F.; Wang, H.W.; Chen, H.Y.; Huang, G.T.; Peng, C.Y. Changes in liver stiffness measurement using acoustic radiation force impulse elastography after antiviral therapy in patients with chronic hepatitis C. *PLoS ONE* **2018**, *13*, e0190455. [CrossRef] [PubMed]

39. Wang, J.H.; Changchien, C.S.; Hung, C.H.; Tung, W.C.; Kee, K.M.; Chen, C.H.; Hu, T.H.; Lee, C.M.; Lu, S.N. Liver stiffness decrease after effective antiviral therapy in patients with chronic hepatitis C: Longitudinal study using FibroScan. *J. Gastroenterol. Hepatol.* **2010**, *25*, 964–969. [CrossRef] [PubMed]

40. Salmon, D.; Dabis, F.; Wittkop, L.; Esterle, L.; Sogni, P.; Trimoulet, P.; Izopet, J.; Serfaty, L.; Paradis, V.; Spire, B.; et al. Regression of liver stiffness after sustained hepatitis C virus (HCV) virological responses among HIV/HCV-coinfected patients. *AIDS* **2015**, *29*, 1821–1830.

41. Elsharkawy, A.; Alem, S.A.; Fouad, R.; El Raziky, M.; El Akel, W.; Abdo, M.; Tantawi, O.; AbdAllah, M.; Bourliere, M.; Esmat, G. Changes in liver stiffness measurements and fibrosis scores following sofosbuvir based treatment regimens without interferon. *J. Gastroenterol. Hepatol.* **2017**, *32*, 1624–1630. [CrossRef] [PubMed]

42. Tachi, Y.; Hirai, T.; Kojima, Y.; Miyata, A.; Ohara, K.; Ishizu, Y.; Honda, T.; Kuzuya, T.; Hayashi, K.; Ishigami, M.; et al. Liver stiffness measurement using acoustic radiation force impulse elastography in hepatitis C virus-infected patients with a sustained virological response. *Aliment. Pharmacol. Ther.* **2016**, *44*, 346–355. [CrossRef] [PubMed]

43. Procopet, B.; Cristea, V.M.; Robic, M.A.; Grigorescu, M.; Agachi, P.S.; Metivier, S.; Peron, J.M.; Selves, J.; Stefanescu, H.; Berzigotti, A.; et al. Serum tests, liver stiffness and artificial neural networks for diagnosing cirrhosis and portal hypertension. *Dig. Liver Dis.* **2015**, *47*, 411–416. [CrossRef] [PubMed]

44. Wong, G.L. Non-invasive assessments for liver fibrosis: The crystal ball we long for. *J. Gastroenterol. Hepatol.* **2018**. [CrossRef] [PubMed]

45. Manousou, P.; Burroughs, A.K.; Tsochatzis, E.; Isgro, G.; Hall, A.; Green, A.; Calvaruso, V.; Ma, G.L.; Gale, J.; Burgess, G.; et al. Digital image analysis of collagen assessment of progression of fibrosis in recurrent HCV after liver transplantation. *J. Hepatol.* **2013**, *58*, 962–968. [CrossRef] [PubMed]

46. Cabassa, P.; Ravanelli, M.; Rossini, A.; Contessi, G.; Almajdalawi, R.; Maroldi, R. Acoustic radiation force impulse quantification of spleen elasticity for assessing liver fibrosis. *Abdom. Imaging* **2015**, *40*, 738–744. [CrossRef] [PubMed]

47. Hézode, C.; Castéra, L.; Roudot-Thoraval, F.; Bouvier-Alias, M.; Rosa, I.; Roulot, D.; Leroy, V.; Mallat, A.; Pawlotsky, J.M. Liver stiffness diminishes with antiviral response in chronic hepatitis C. *Aliment. Pharmacol. Ther.* **2011**, *34*, 656–663. [CrossRef] [PubMed]

48. Stasi, C.; Arena, U.; Zignego, A.L.; Corti, G.; Monti, M.; Triboli, E.; Pellegrini, E.; Renzo, S.; Leoncini, L.; Marra, F.; et al. Longitudinal assessment of liver stiffness in patients undergoing antiviral treatment for hepatitis C. *Dig. Liver Dis.* **2013**, *45*, 840–843. [CrossRef] [PubMed]

49. Łucejko, M.; Flisiak, R. Effect of HCV core antigen and RNA clearance during therapy with direct-acting antivirals on hepatic stiffness measured with shear wave elastography in patients with chronic viral hepatitis C. *Appl. Sci.* **2018**, *8*, 198. [CrossRef]

50. Chon, Y.E.; Park, J.Y.; Myoung, S.M.; Jung, K.S.; Kim, B.K.; Kim, S.U.; Kim, D.Y.; Ahn, S.H.; Han, K.H. Improvement of liver fibrosis after long-term antiviral therapy assessed by Fibroscan in chronic hepatitis B patients with advanced fibrosis. *Am. J. Gastroenterol.* **2017**, *112*, 882–891. [CrossRef] [PubMed]

51. Fung, J.; Lai, C.L.; Wong, D.K.; Seto, W.K.; Hung, I.; Yuen, M.F. Significant changes in liver stiffness measurements in patients with chronic hepatitis B: 3-year follow-up study. *J. Viral Hepat.* **2011**, *18*, e200–e205. [CrossRef] [PubMed]

52. Ogawa, E.; Furusyo, N.; Murata, M.; Ohnishi, H.; Toyoda, K.; Taniai, H.; Ihara, T.; Ikezaki, H.; Hayashi, T.; Kainuma, M.; et al. Longitudinal assessment of liver stiffness by transient elastography for chronic hepatitis B patients treated with nucleoside analog. *Hepatol. Res.* **2011**, *41*, 1178–1188. [CrossRef] [PubMed]

53. Kim, J.K.; Ma, D.W.; Lee, K.S.; Paik, Y.H. Assessment of hepatic fibrosis regression by transient elastography in patients with chronic hepatitis B treated with oral antiviral agents. *J. Korean Med. Sci.* **2014**, *29*, 570–575. [CrossRef] [PubMed]

54. Li, X.; Jin, Q.; Zhang, H.; Jing, X.; Ding, Z.; Zhou, H.; Zhang, Z.; Yan, D.; Li, D.; Gao, P.; et al. Changes in liver stiffness and its associated factors during oral antiviral therapy in Chinese patients with chronic hepatitis B. *Exp. Ther. Med.* **2017**, *13*, 1169–1175. [CrossRef] [PubMed]

55. Rinaldi, L.; Ascione, A.; Messina, V.; Rosato, V.; Valente, G.; Sangiovanni, V.; Zampino, R.; Marrone, A.; Fontanella, L.; de Rosa, N.; et al. Influence of antiviral therapy on the liver stiffness in chronic HBV hepatitis. *Infection* **2018**, *46*, 231–238. [CrossRef] [PubMed]

56. Li, Q.; Chen, L.; Zhou, Y. Changes of FibroScan, APRI, and FIB-4 in chronic hepatitis B patients with significant liver histological changes receiving 3-year entecavir therapy. *Clin. Exp. Med.* **2018**. [CrossRef] [PubMed]

57. Qiu, T.; Wang, H.; Song, J.; Guo, G.; Shi, Y.; Luo, Y.; Liu, J. Could ultrasound elastography reflect liver function? *Ultrasound Med. Biol.* **2018**, *44*, 779–785. [CrossRef] [PubMed]

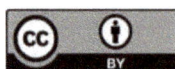

© 2018 by the authors. Licensee MDPI, Basel, Switzerland. This article is an open access article distributed under the terms and conditions of the Creative Commons Attribution (CC BY) license (http://creativecommons.org/licenses/by/4.0/).

applied
sciences

MDPI

Article

Quantitative Analysis of Patellar Tendon Abnormality in Asymptomatic Professional "Pallapugno" Players: A Texture-Based Ultrasound Approach

Kristen M. Meiburger [1,*], Massimo Salvi [1] , Maurizio Giacchino [2], U. Rajendra Acharya [3,4,5], Marco A. Minetto [6], Cristina Caresio [7] and Filippo Molinari [1]

[1] Biolab, Department of Electronics and Telecomunications, Politecnico di Torino, 10129 Turin, Italy; massimo.salvi@polito.it (M.S.); filippo.molinari@polito.it (F.M.)
[2] Medical Lab, 14100 Asti, Italy; calcki@alice.it
[3] Department of Electronics and Computer Engineering, Ngee Ann Polytechnic, Singapore 599489, Singapore; Rajendra_Udyavara_ACHARYA@np.edu.sg
[4] Department of Biomedical Engineering, School of Science and Technology, Singapore University of Social Sciences, Singapore 599484, Singapore
[5] Department of Biomedical Engineering, Faculty of Engineering, University of Malaya, Kuala Lumpur 50603, Malaysia
[6] Division of Physical Medicine and Rehabilitation, Department of Surgical Sciences, University of Turin, 10126 Turin, Italy; marco.minetto@unito.it
[7] Cardiovascular Biomechanics, Department of Biomedical Engineering, Eindhoven University of Technology, 5600 MB Eindhoven, The Netherlands; c.caresio@tue.nl
* Correspondence: kristen.meiburger@polito.it; Tel.: +39-011-090-4207

Received: 30 March 2018; Accepted: 23 April 2018; Published: 25 April 2018

Featured Application: Quantitative texture analysis of tendon ultrasound images for determination of subclinical tendinopathy.

Abstract: Abnormalities in B-mode ultrasound images of the patellar tendon often take place in asymptomatic athletes but it is still not clear if these modifications forego or can predict the development of tendinopathy. Subclinical tendinopathy can be arbitrarily defined as either (1) the presence of light structural changes in B-mode ultrasound images in association with mild neovascularization (determined with Power Doppler images) or (2) the presence of moderate/severe structural changes with or without neovascularization. Up to now, the structural changes and neovascularization of the tendon are evaluated qualitatively by visual inspection of ultrasound images. The aim of this study is to investigate the capability of a quantitative texture-based approach to determine tendon abnormality of "pallapugno" players. B-mode ultrasound images of the patellar tendon were acquired in 14 players and quantitative texture parameters were calculated within a Region of Interest (ROI) of both the non-dominant and the dominant tendon. A total of 90 features were calculated for each ROI, including 6 first-order descriptors, 24 Haralick features, and 60 higher-order spectra and entropy features. These features on the dominant and non-dominant side were used to perform a multivariate linear regression analysis (MANOVA) and our results show that the descriptors can be effectively used to determine tendon abnormality and, more importantly, the occurrence of subclinical tendinopathy.

Keywords: ultrasonography; tendinopathy; texture analysis; quantitative

---

1. Introduction

Ultrasonography is an effective non-invasive imaging technique used in musculoskeletal medicine both for (1) investigating the skeletal muscle structure and calculating quantitative muscle parameters [1–4] and for (2) qualitative and quantitative assessment of tendon structure (echo-intensity) and size (thickness, length, and cross-sectional area) [5–8]. Ultrasound imaging presents many advantages, including the fact that it is portable, has low associated costs, is non-invasive, and does not use any ionizing radiation for imaging, but rather innocuous high frequency sound waves. On the other hand, however, it is a very operator-dependent technique and presents a high intra- and inter-reader variability [9].

Ultrasound imaging of the patellar tendon is commonly employed to study tendon abnormalities that could occur because of repetitive overload, which is a common happening in professional athletes of various disciplines [10–13]. Patellar tendinopathy (PT) is especially common in athletes that play sports that require jumping, such as basketball and volleyball, giving it its common-term name of "jumper's knee" [14,15]. Recent studies focused on the analysis of changes in elastic properties of the patellar tendon using shear wave imaging [16–21]. Zhang et al. [18] showed that athletes with unilateral PT had a stiffer tendon (i.e., higher shear elastic modulus) on the non-painful side when compared to the painful side (25.8 ± 10.6 kPa vs. 43.6 ± 17.9 kPa, respectively), whereas healthy controls showed no difference of stiffness between sides (27.5 ± 11.3 kPa vs. 27.9 ± 8.4 kPa). In their study, they also conducted a morphological analysis and found that the athletes with PT had a larger painful tendon compared with the contralateral non-painful side (thickness: 6.9 ± 1.8 mm vs. 4.6 ± 0.6 mm, respectively), whereas the controls had no difference between sides (5.6 ± 1.2 mm vs. 5.3 ± 1.0 mm). Morphological abnormalities in the tendon ultrasound image, such as increased tendon thickness, neovascularization, and presence of hypoechoic areas, have also been found in a large percentage of asymptomatic athletes [9,11,13,22]. Recently, Giacchino et al. [23] also conducted a study of patellar tendon size and structure in throwers and found that the prevalence of subclinical tendinopathy was high in the non-dominant patellar tendon as a possible result of the repeated non-dominant lower limb overload. To do so, the authors arbitrarily defined subclinical tendinopathy as "the presence of either light structural changes in association with at least mild neovascularization or moderate/severe structural changes with/without neovascularization" [23]. In the study, however, the determination of structural changes was done by quantitative assessments of tendon echo intensity and size and by qualitative analysis of the B-mode ultrasound images of both the dominant and non-dominant side, which is a very subjective technique and can depend greatly on the ultrasound scanner settings [24]. On the contrary, texture features that can be calculated on the B-mode ultrasound image are intensity-invariant and have proven to be informative in the characterization of various tissues, such as breast [25], ovarian tumors [26], thyroid lesions [27], liver [28], and recently also in musculoskeletal images [29].

In this study, we aim to quantitatively analyze the presence of patellar tendon abnormality and subclinical tendinopathy in professional asymptomatic players using a texture-based morphological approach and the same image database as presented in [23]. In particular, the study provides quantitative texture features calculated on the images initially used for the determination of a qualitative structure score [23], and analyzes the capability of this approach to discriminate between the dominant and non-dominant side of the player, and to determine the presence of subclinical tendinopathy as defined previously.

2. Materials and Methods

2.1. Subject Database

Fourteen elite players of "pallapugno" who did not present any neuromuscular or skeletal impairment volunteered to participate in the study. This sport is similar to Frisian handball and implies that throwers repeatedly overload the non-dominant lower limb. The mean age was 21.8 ± 4.2 years and all participants were male. Side dominance was determined using the "Waterloo Handedness and Footedness Questionnaires—Revised" [30], according to which, all subjects were right side dominant. The study conformed to the guidelines of the Declaration of Helsinki and was approved by the local ethics committee of the University of Turin. A detailed explanation of the protocol was given to the participants who then gave written informed consent before participating.

2.2. Ultrasound Image Acquisition and Protocol

The subjects were asked to refrain from performing any strenuous physical activity 24 h before the experimental session, during which B-mode ultrasound patellar tendon images were acquired. Both the dominant and the non-dominant side were studied. The same experienced sonographer (M.G.) performed all image acquisitions, for a total of 20 images for each subject. Specifically, while the subject had the quadriceps muscle relaxed and was lying in a supine position, 8 images were acquired with a knee angle of 30°, and then with a knee angle of 0°, 12 scans were acquired. For the purpose of this texture-analysis study, 6 images on each side were analyzed as reported in Table 1. The remaining 4 images on each side were employed also for qualitative assessments of neovascularization and tendon structure as reported in [23]. According to the definition as cited in the Introduction [23], 5 subjects out of the 14 were found to be affected by subclinical tendinopathy (i.e., 5 subjects demonstrated the presence of light structural changes in association with at least mild neovascularization or moderate/severe structural changes with/without neovascularization).

Table 1. Tendon B-mode image acquisition protocol for dominant and non-dominant side.

Plane	Probe Position	Knee Angle
Transversal	Proximal	0°
Longitudinal	Proximal	0°
Transversal	Proximal	30°
Longitudinal	Proximal	30°
Transversal	Central	30°
Longitudinal	Central	30°

All images were acquired using a ClearVue 550 ultrasound machine (Philips Medical Systems, Milan, Italy) equipped with a linear array transducer (Philips L12-5, central frequency = 5–12 MHz). The time-gain compensation was kept equal for all scans (neutral), dynamic image compression was turned off, and the gain was set at 50% of the total range. The image acquisition preset was kept the same for each subject and throughout the study. The ultrasound images were stored as DICOM files and analyzed offline.

2.3. Texture Feature Extraction

All images were visually inspected and analyzed by the same experienced operator (C.C.) who drew a region of interest (ROI) encompassing the tendon area within the ultrasound image frame. Figure 1 shows some examples of ROIs for one subject, comparing the dominant and non-dominant side of the tendon. Figure 2 displays some example images of the non-dominant side of the players, highlighting the difference between a subject with a "normal" tendon structure and a subject with an abnormal tendon structure. An abnormal tendon structure was taken as one that fell into the category of subclinical tendinopathy as arbitrarily defined in the study by Giacchino et al. [23] and as stated previously.

Numerous texture features were then extracted from within the ROI of each image, including both the dominant side and the non-dominant side of the player. Specifically, a total of 90 texture features were extracted for each ROI, for a total of 1080 textures features extracted for each subject (90 features × 6 images × 2 sides). The texture features can be divided into the following three main categories: (1) first-order statistical descriptors, (2) Haralick features, and (3) higher-order spectra, entropy features, and Hu's moments, which are subsequently described in more detail. All texture parameters were calculated by custom developed software in MATLAB (The MathWorks, Natick, MA, USA).

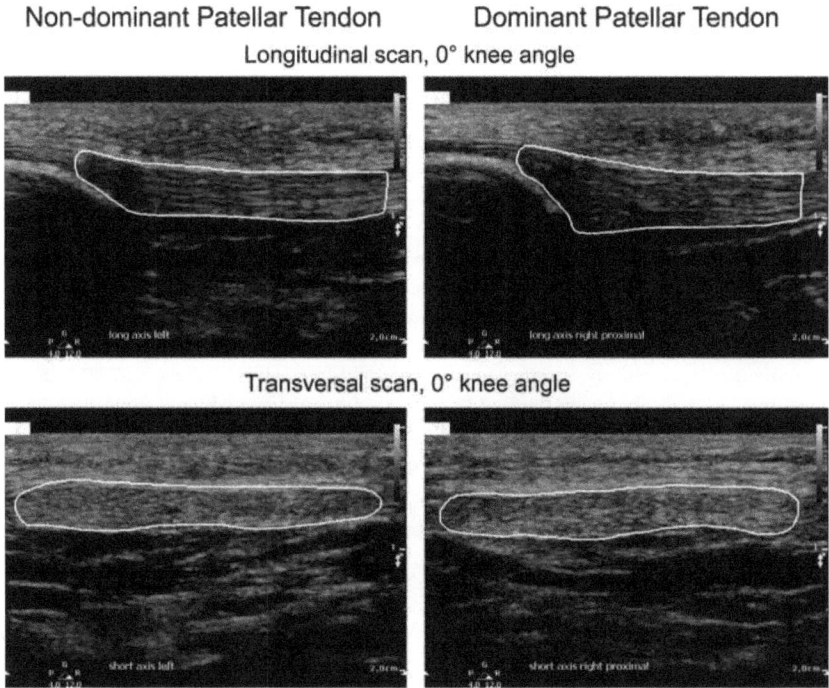

Figure 1. Representative patellar tendon images of one player displaying both the dominant and non-dominant side.

2.3.1. First-Order Statistical Descriptors

Six texture features that are based on the first order statistics were extracted: pixel intensity mean, variance, standard deviation, skewness, kurtosis, and energy. These features depend on the single gray level of the pixel and the mathematical descriptions are defined in Table 2.

Table 2. Mathematical description of first-order statistical features.

Feature Name	Mathematical Description
Mean (m)	$m = \sum_{x=1}^{M} \sum_{y=1}^{N} \dfrac{I(x,y)}{M \times N}$
Standard deviation (σ)	$\sigma = \sqrt{\dfrac{\sum_{x=1}^{M} \sum_{y=1}^{N} \{I(x,y) - m\}^2}{M \times N}}$
Variance (σ^2)	$\sigma^2 = \dfrac{\sum_{x=1}^{M} \sum_{y=1}^{N} \{I(x,y) - m\}^2}{M \times N}$
Skewness (S_k)	$S_k = \dfrac{1}{M \times N} \dfrac{\sum_{x=1}^{M} \sum_{y=1}^{N} \{I(x,y) - m\}^3}{\sigma^3}$
Kurtosis (K_t)	$K_t = \dfrac{1}{M \times N} \dfrac{\sum_{x=1}^{M} \sum_{y=1}^{N} \{I(x,y) - m\}^4}{\sigma^4}$
Energy$_1$ (E_1)	$E_1 = \sum_{x=1}^{M} \sum_{y=1}^{N} I(x,y)^2$

$I(x,y)$ denotes the input muscle ROI.

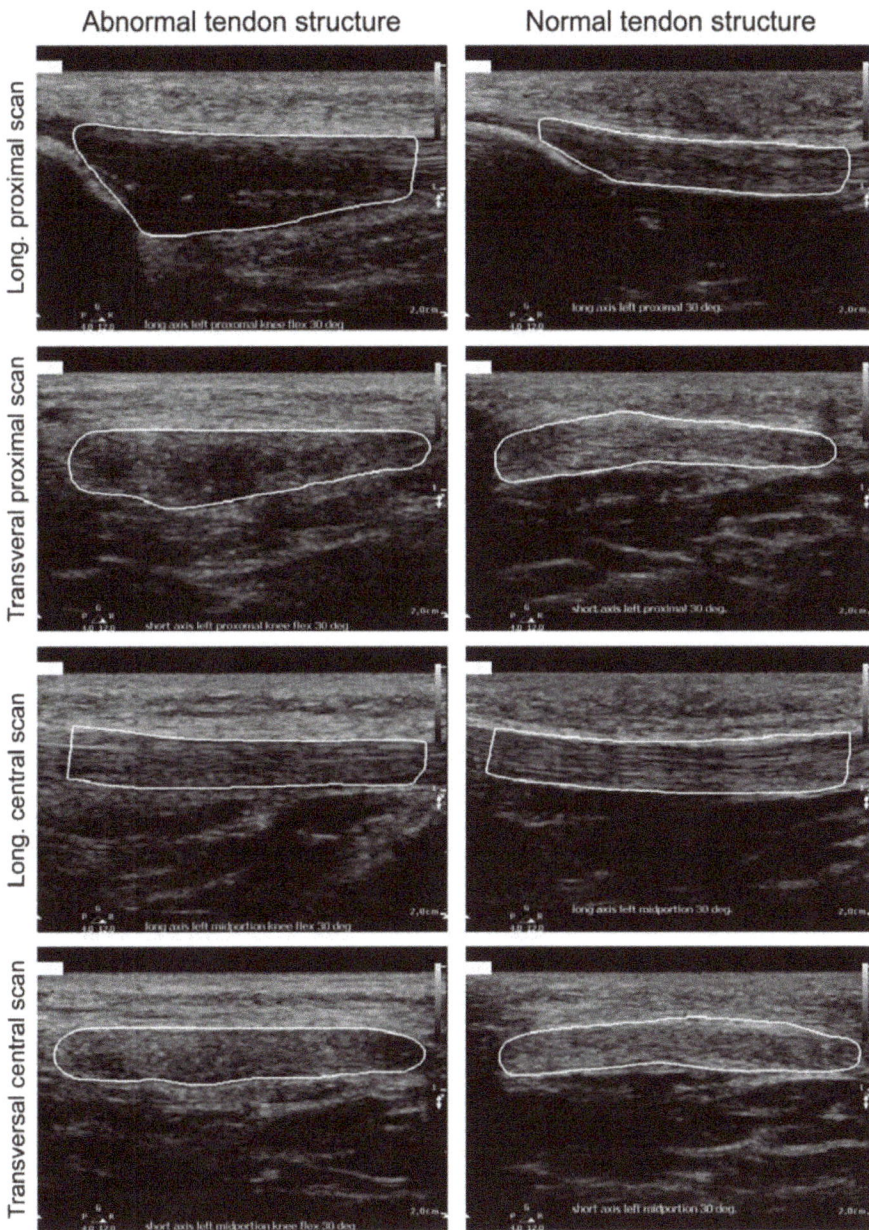

Figure 2. Representative patellar tendon images showing the non-dominant side of two players, one with a normal tendon structure (**right panels**), and one player with an abnormal tendon structure (**left panels**). An abnormal tendon structure was taken as one that fell into the category of subclinical tendinopathy as arbitrarily defined in the study by Giacchino et al. [23]. All scans reported in the figure were acquired with the knee at a 30° position. Long: longitudinal.

2.3.2. Haralick Features

The Haralick features are based on the gray level co-occurrence matrix (GCLM) [31], which measures the number of times a specific intensity pattern between adjacent pixels is repeated. Since adjacency can be measured in four principal directions (e.g., vertical, horizontal, and two diagonal directions), the GLCM is computed using four angles: $0°$, $45°$, $90°$, and $135°$. The Haralick features mathematically describe the GLCM through the calculation of the symmetry, contrast, homogeneity, entropy, energy, and correlation. These features are computed for four directions, so a total of 24 descriptors are extracted for each ROI. The mathematical description of these features can be found in Table 3.

Table 3. Mathematical description of Haralick features.

Feature Name	Mathematical Description
Symmetry (I_{sym})	$I_{sym} = 1 - \sum_{i=0}^{N-1} \sum_{j=0}^{N-1} \lvert i - j \rvert P(i,j)$
Contrast (I_{con})	$I_{con} = \sum_{n=0}^{N-1} n^2 \left\{ \sum_{i=0}^{N} \sum_{j=0}^{N-1} P(i,j) \right\}$
Homogeneity (I_{hmg})	$I_{hmg} = \sum_{i=0}^{N-1} \sum_{j=0}^{N-1} \dfrac{1}{1 + (i-j)^2} P(i,j)$
Entropy (I_{Entr})	$I_{Entr} = -\sum_{i=0}^{N-1} \sum_{j=0}^{N-1} P(i,j) \log P(i,j)$
Energy (I_{Enrg})	$I_{Enrg} = \sum_{i=0}^{N-1} \sum_{j=0}^{N-1} P(i,j)^2$
Correlation (I_{cor})	$I_{cor} = \dfrac{\sum_{i=0}^{N-1} \sum_{j=0}^{N-1} (i,j)P(i,j) - \mu_x \mu_y}{\sigma_x \sigma_y}$

$\sigma_x, \sigma_y, \mu_y, \mu_y$ are the standard deviations and means of P_x, P_y, which are the partial probability density functions. $p_x(i) = i$th entry in the marginal-probability matrix obtained by summing the rows of $P(i,j)$.

2.3.3. Higher-Order Spectra, Entropy Features, and Hu's Moments

Higher-order spectra (HOS) invariants were first extracted from each ROI, which retains both phase and magnitude information of the image [32]. The normalized bispectrum and phase entropies are calculated from bispectrum plots for every $20°$ (i.e., 9 directions, from $0°$ to $160°$), generating a total of 45 features since each bispectrum plot can be described with 5 features [32]. To further analyze and measure pixel variations, the energy, Shannon [33], Renyi [34], Fuzzy [35], Kapur [36], Yager [37], Vajda [38], and maximum entropy [39] were calculated on each ROI. Finally, 7 Hu's moments which represent the invariant patterns of the image were extracted [40].

2.4. Statistical Analysis

The overall number of texture features for each ROI was equal to 90, and each subject was represented by 6 different B-mode images on both the dominant and non-dominant side. We used a multivariate analysis of variance (MANOVA) to test the equality of the means among groups, considering both the discrimination between (1) dominant side texture features and non-dominant side texture features, and (2) subclinical tendinopathy texture features and non-subclinical tendinopathy texture features, considering only the non-dominant side. In order to avoid singularities in the observation matrix, collinear variables were first removed by the Belsley collinearity diagnostics technique [41] prior to the MANOVA analysis. The default value of tolerance for the Belsley collinearity diagnostics was used (tolerance value = 0.5) when considering the discrimination between the dominant and non-dominant side. On the other hand, when determining the presence or absence of subclinical tendinopathy, a tolerance value of 0.35 was used. These optimal values were employed since a higher tolerance value led to an insufficient removal of collinear variables, whereas a lower value discarded an excessive number of variables.

The dimension of the MANOVA was used to assess how many groups the data belongs to; in particular, a dimension equal to 0 means that it is not possible to reject the null hypothesis that all subjects belong to the same group. Similarly, a dimension equal to 1 indicates that we can reject the null hypothesis, meaning that the subjects can be divided into two groups. The Receiving Operator Characteristic (ROC) analysis [42] was then performed on the first canonical variable in order to test the classification quality obtained with the MANOVA analysis.

3. Results

3.1. Comparison between Dominant and Non-Dominant Side

When the tendon side (dominant or non-dominant) was considered as the dependent variable, 28 collinear variables were removed using the Belsley collinearity diagnostics technique, therefore leaving a final total of 62 texture features that were considered in the MANOVA analysis. The MANOVA dimension of the groups means was equal to 1 ($p < 0.05$). MANOVA dimensionality is fundamental for understanding how the different samples were distributed on the canonical variables hyperplane. In fact, MANOVA canonical variables are linear combinations of the original texture features and are constructed so as to maximize the variance among groups. Finding a dimension of 1 therefore ensures that one canonical variable (i.e., the first, since they are ordered with decreasing explained variance) is sufficient to discriminate between tendon images of the dominant side of the players or of the non-dominant side of the players. Figure 3a shows the plot of the samples based on the first and second canonical variable, where a full dark circle indicates the dominant side of the player, and the full light gray circle indicates the non-dominant side. As can be seen in this figure, the first canonical variable is able to discriminate between the dominant and non-dominant side of the players.

The first column of Table 4 lists the texture features that had the highest absolute weight on the first canonical variable, meaning that they were the most discriminant for the determination of the side. The ROC analysis gave an area under the curve (AUC) equal to 0.906 (Figure 3b). Considering an optimal threshold as the one determined by the maximum Youden index (sensitivity + specificity − 1), the final classification results gave a sensitivity equal to 86.9%, a specificity equal to 79.8%, and an accuracy equal to 83.3%.

Table 4. Image features that were the most discriminant between dominant and non-dominant side (all subjects and only healthy subjects) and to determine subclinical tendinopathy.

Most Discriminant Features for Side Determination (Weight)		Most Discriminant Features for Side Determination (Only Healthy Subjects) (Weight)		Most Discriminant Features for Subclinical Tendinopathy Determination (Weight)	
Kurtosis	(−65.0)	H. Homogeneity (45°)	(172.0)	H. Symmetry (0°)	(−24.5)
H. Correlation (0°)	(58.9)	H. Contrast (45°)	(−155.8)	H. Contrast (45°)	(−14.3)
H. Contrast (0°)	(12.9)	H. Symmetry (45°)	(−48.7)	H. Entropy (0°)	(14.2)
Skewness	(−12.3)	H. Symmetry (0°)	(−29.7)	H. Correlation (45°)	(13.4)
H. Entropy (0°)	(9.6)	H. Energy (0°)	(27.2)	H. Homogeneity (0°)	(5.5)
H. Correlation (45°)	(7.0)	H. Correlation (0°)	(27.1)	Mean Intensity	(4.8)
H. Energy (45°)	(−6.3)	H. Correlation (135°)	(6.1)	First−order Entropy	(4.3)
H. Homogeneity (0°)	(3.5)	H. Energy (45°)	(−5.3)	Kurtosis	(−4.2)
H. Entropy (45°)	(2.3)	Mean Intensity	(5.1)	Variance	(3.0)
H. Symmetry (45°)	(−2.2)	H. Entropy (45°)	(4.8)	H. Correlation (0°)	(2.9)

Furthermore, we then analyzed the same dependent variable (dominant or non-dominant side) but removing the subjects that presented subclinical tendinopathy. This further analysis was done to ensure that the presence of these subjects did not skew the previous results. In this case, 16 collinear variables were removed, leaving a final total of 74 texture features that were considered in the MANOVA analysis. Figure 3c shows the plot of the samples based on the first and second canonical variable, where a full dark circle indicates the dominant side of the player, and the full light gray circle indicates the non-dominant side. As can be seen in this figure, the first canonical variable is again able to discriminate between the dominant and non-dominant side of the healthy players.

The second column of Table 4 lists the texture features that had the highest absolute weight on the first canonical variable, meaning that they were the most discriminant for the determination of the side. The ROC analysis gave an area under the curve (AUC) equal to 0.989 (Figure 3d). Considering an optimal threshold as the one determined by the maximum Youden index, the final classification results gave sensitivity, specificity, and accuracy all equal to 96.3%.

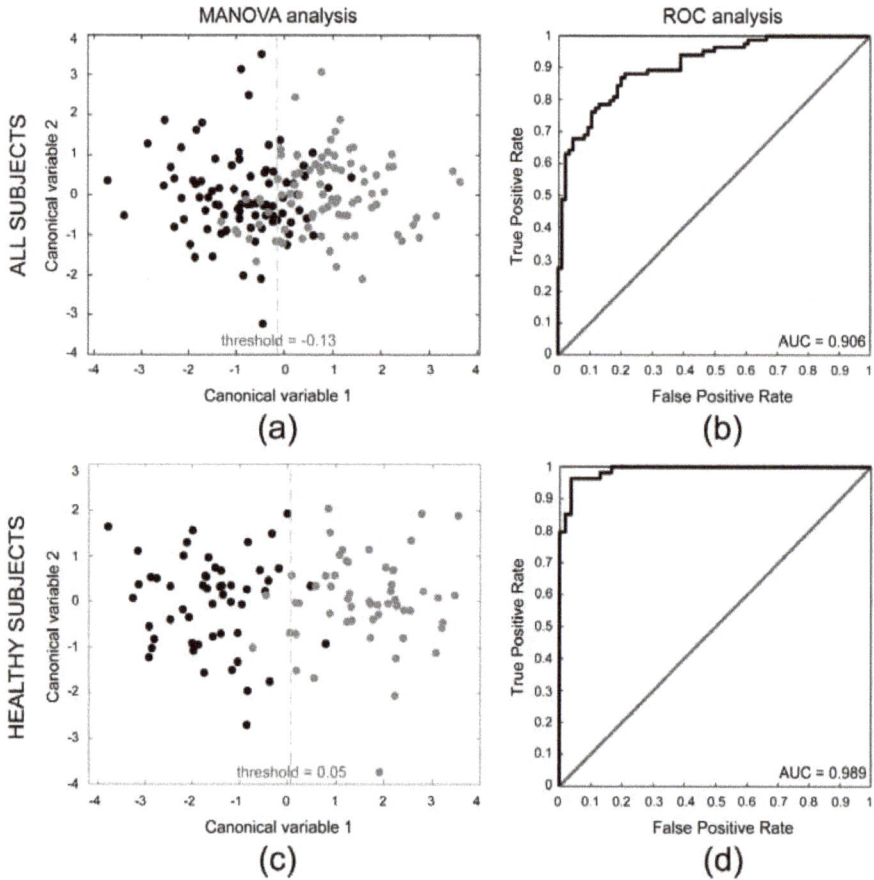

Figure 3. Results obtained when comparing dominant and non-dominant side texture features considering all subjects (**first row**) and only subjects with normal tendon structure (**second row**). The black circles represent the dominant side textures features, while the gray circles represent the non-dominant side texture features. (**a**) Representation of all subjects in the plane of the first two canonical variables obtained by a MANOVA analysis. The vertical gray dotted line represents the optimal threshold used (maximum Youden index) to obtain the sensitivity (86.9%), specificity (79.8%), and accuracy (83.3%) results; (**b**) ROC analysis results demonstrating the classification quality of the first MANOVA canonical variable, with an AUC equal to 0.906; (**c**) Representation of the healthy subjects in the plane of the first two canonical variables obtained by a MANOVA analysis. The vertical gray dotted line represents the optimal threshold used (maximum Youden index) to obtain the sensitivity (96.3%), specificity (96.3%), and accuracy (96.3%) results; (**d**) ROC analysis results demonstrating the classification quality of the first MANOVA canonical variable, with an AUC equal to 0.989.

3.2. Comparison between Subclinical Tendinopathy and Non-Subclinical Tendinopathy

When aiming to discriminate between the patients that presented subclinical tendinopathy and those that did not, and using only the images acquired on the non-dominant side of each player (i.e., a non-dominant PT is expected in the investigated group of thrower players given that the throwing performance of these players implies a repeated overload of the non-dominant lower limb), 54 collinear variables were removed using the Belsley collinearity diagnostics technique, therefore leaving a final total of 36 texture features that were considered in the MANOVA analysis. The MANOVA analysis again showed a dimension of the groups means equal to 1 ($p < 0.05$). We can therefore be assured that the first canonical variable is able to discriminate between these two cases, as can be seen also in Figure 4a. In this figure, the full gray circles represent the "healthy" cases, whereas the black circles represent the subclinical tendinopathy cases.

The second column of Table 4 lists the texture features that had the highest weight on the first canonical variable, meaning that they were the most discriminant for the determination of subclinical tendinopathy. The ROC analysis gave forth an area under the curve (AUC) equal to 0.967 (Figure 4b). Considering an optimal threshold as the one determined by the maximum Youden index, the final classification results gave a sensitivity equal to 93.3%, a specificity equal to 90.7%, and an accuracy equal to 91.7%.

As can be appreciated from Table 4, the first-order and Haralick features proved to be the most discriminant for both determining the dominant or non-dominant side and in determining the presence or absence of subclinical tendinopathy. The higher-order spectra and entropy features, on the other hand, were not among the 10 most discriminant features.

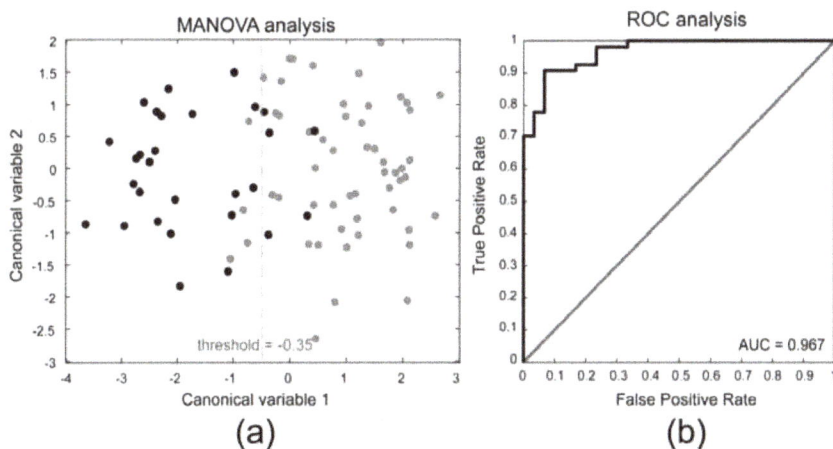

Figure 4. Results obtained when comparing subjects with ($n = 5$) and without subclinical tendinopathy ($n = 9$). (**a**) Representation of the subjects in the plane of the first two canonical variables obtained by a MANOVA analysis. The black circles represent the texture features of subjects with subclinical tendinopathy, while the gray circles represent the texture features of subjects without subclinical tendinopathy. The vertical gray dotted line represents the optimal threshold (maximum Youden index) used to obtain the sensitivity (93.3%), specificity (90.7%), and accuracy (91.7%) results; (**b**) ROC analysis results demonstrating the classification quality of the first MANOVA canonical variable, with an AUC equal to 0.967.

4. Discussion

In the present study, quantitative ultrasonography was performed in tendon images of 14 players acquired on both the dominant and non-dominant side. Ninety texture features were calculated in the tendon region of each image in order assess the characterization performance of the texture descriptors in discriminating between sides and in discriminating the presence or absence of subclinical tendinopathy, as arbitrarily defined. Our results show that the first-order and Haralick features proved to be highly linked to both tendon side and the presence of subclinical tendinopathy, whereas the higher-order spectra and entropy features did not add any further information when considering these two cases. To the best of our knowledge, this is the first study that used texture features for the quantitative analysis of tendon images for the determination of patellar tendon abnormality.

The tendinopathic process includes an increase in the number of vessels, tendon thickness, hydrated components of the extracellular matrix, and the disorganization of collagen fibers and breakdown of tissue organization [43–46]. Most of these findings may underlie the occurrence of ultrasound markers of tendon histopathology, such as increased tendon cross-sectional area and vascularity and decreased tendon echogenicity and stiffness. In fact, PT can also be investigated through the employment of ultrasonic shear wave imaging [18,21,47–49], which gives information about the stiffness of the affected tendon, but it is still typically evaluated through the ultrasonographic assessment of tendon structure and size, such as the presence of hypoechoic areas, altered vascularity, and localized tendon thickening. A previous study by the authors demonstrated quantitatively how tendon size and echogenicity were related to the presence of subclinical tendinopathy [23]. However, in the study, only a qualitative analysis was done to assess structural changes and the presence of neovascularization. In this current study, we showed how we can effectively discriminate subjects based solely on the quantitative texture features.

As can be noted, the Haralick features were quite determinant in understanding if an image was either of the dominant or non-dominant side of the player and also in discriminating between the presence or absence of subclinical tendinopathy. These features are based on statistics calculated on the gray level co-occurrence matrix, which describes the patterns of neighboring pixels in an image, giving an idea of the complexity of the various distributions of pixel intensity. Although no histological analysis was done in this study, we can hypothesize that these features can be attributed to a disorganization of collagen fibers and breakdown of tissue organization which are typically not assessable through a mere calculation of tendon size or the presence of hypoechoic areas. It can be noted how the most discriminant features are different when considering side determination when including or excluding the subclinical tendinopathy subjects. In fact, when these subjects are included, the "kurtosis" and "skewness" features are among the most discriminant. These two features measure how outlier-prone a distribution is and the asymmetry of the data distribution, respectively, showing how, while the MANOVA analysis is still able to correctly discriminate between dominant and non-dominant sides, the subclinical tendinopathy subjects present discriminative features that are more related to a disorganization of tissues. This can also be observed when discriminating between subjects with and without subclinical tendinopathy, where the Haralick Symmetry feature (0°) is the most discriminant feature, and where numerous other features that can describe the tissue organization (such as entropy, correlation, homogeneity) are also found to be discriminant. As can be noted in the second column of Table 4, when considering only subjects without subclinical tendinopathy and discriminating the side determination, the first two features (Homogeneity and Contrast) represent a very high weight, approximately three times higher than the third feature. From this analysis, we can see that even when considering only healthy subjects, there is still a net difference in the tendon ultrasound texture parameters that relate to tissue organization and echogenicity, which is also in accordance with the study by Giacchino et al. [23].

A main finding of this study is how, through a quantitative textural analysis of only B-mode images, it is possible to determine with high accuracy the subjects that presented a subclinical tendinopathy as defined arbitrarily by inspecting both B-mode images and Power Doppler images (for the assessment of neovascularization). We can therefore hypothesize that a quantitative texture-based approach as presented here can be of aid for the diagnosis (as well as monitoring and prognosis) of subclinical tendinopathy in a standardized manner, requiring only the identification of the tendon ROI within the B-mode image.

The clinical management of patellar tendinopathy is currently complicated as the diagnosis is currently based on a combination of clinical criteria and ultrasound/MRI findings. However, there are no means to detect the onset of tendinopathy before the appearance of clinical signs and no tools are currently available for the prediction and prognosis of patellar tendinopathy. Therefore, the availability of ultrasound markers of tendon histopathology can be useful to track the progression of tendinopathy over time and may help to indicate early response to therapeutic interventions.

However, further studies are required to establish a causal association between ultrasound markers of tendon histopathology and the actual development of tendinopathy as well as the increased risk of tendon rupture.

This work has the following main limitations. First of all, the sample size was small and included only athletes that played a very specific sport, making it difficult to generalize our findings to other populations. Secondly, no histopathological assessment was done to confirm the development of tendinopathy.

In the future, we plan to extend our work presented here and analyze the potential correlations between tendon texture features and its stiffness, and to develop an automated tool for the segmentation of the tendon in the ultrasound frame, which would enhance both the morphological and elastic analysis of tendon properties.

5. Conclusions

In conclusion, the current study confirmed the possibility of identifying tendon abnormalities through the quantitative texture analysis of ultrasound B-mode images. Specifically, we showed how it is possible to both discriminate between the dominant and non-dominant patellar tendon of "pallapugno" players and, more importantly, to discriminate between players with or without subclinical tendinopathy by using only the quantitative texture features calculated on B-mode images, independent of both tendon size and information derived from a Power Doppler analysis.

Author Contributions: F.M. and M.A.M. conceived and designed the experiments; M.G. and C.C. performed the experiments; K.M.M. and M.S. analyzed the data; U.R.A. contributed analysis tools; K.M.M., F.M., M.A.M. and U.R.A. wrote the paper.

Conflicts of Interest: The authors declare no conflict of interest.

References

1. Pillen, S.; Arts, I.M.P.; Zwarts, M.J. Muscle ultrasound in neuromuscular disorders. *Muscle Nerve* **2008**, *37*, 679–693. [CrossRef] [PubMed]
2. Reeves, N.D.; Maganaris, C.N.; Narici, M.V. Ultrasonographic assessment of human skeletal muscle size. *Eur. J. Appl. Physiol.* **2004**, *91*, 116–118. [CrossRef] [PubMed]
3. Meiburger, K.M.; Acharya, U.R.; Molinari, F. Automated localization and segmentation techniques for B-mode ultrasound images: A review. *Comput. Biol. Med.* **2018**, *92*, 210–235. [CrossRef] [PubMed]
4. Caresio, C.; Salvi, M.; Molinari, F.; Meiburger, K.M.; Minetto, M.A. Fully Automated Muscle Ultrasound Analysis (MUSA): Robust and Accurate Muscle Thickness Measurement. *Ultrasound Med. Biol.* **2017**, *43*, 195–205. [CrossRef] [PubMed]
5. Martinoli, C.; Derchi, L.E.; Pastorino, C.; Bertolotto, M.; Silvestri, E. Analysis of echotexture of tendons with US. *Radiology* **1993**, *186*, 839–843. [CrossRef] [PubMed]
6. Rasmussen, O.S. Sonography of tendons. *Scand. J. Med. Sci. Sports* **2000**, *10*, 360–364. [CrossRef] [PubMed]
7. Fredberg, U.; Bolvig, L.; Andersen, N.; Stengaard-Pedersen, K. Ultrasonography in Evaluation of Achilles and Patella Tendon Thickness. *Eur. J. Ultrasound* **2007**, *29*, 60–65. [CrossRef] [PubMed]
8. Gellhorn, A.C.; Morgenroth, D.C.; Goldstein, B. A Novel Sonographic Method of Measuring Patellar Tendon Length. *Ultrasound Med. Biol.* **2012**, *38*, 719–726. [CrossRef] [PubMed]

9.   Sunding, K.; Fahlström, M.; Werner, S.; Forssblad, M.; Willberg, L. Evaluation of Achilles and patellar tendinopathy with greyscale ultrasound and colour Doppler: Using a four-grade scale. *Knee Surg. Sport Traumatol. Arthrosc.* **2016**, *24*, 1988–1996. [CrossRef] [PubMed]

10. Kulig, K.; Landel, R.; Chang, Y.-J.; Hannanvash, N.; Reischl, S.F.; Song, P.; Bashford, G.R. Patellar tendon morphology in volleyball athletes with and without patellar tendinopathy. *Scand. J. Med. Sci. Sports* **2013**, *23*, e81–e88. [CrossRef] [PubMed]

11. Giombini, A.; Dragoni, S.; Di Cesare, A.; Di Cesare, M.; Del Buono, A.; Maffulli, N. Asymptomatic Achilles, patellar, and quadriceps tendinopathy: A longitudinal clinical and ultrasonographic study in elite fencers. *Scand. J. Med. Sci. Sports* **2013**, *23*, 311–316. [CrossRef] [PubMed]

12. Comin, J.; Cook, J.L.; Malliaras, P.; McCormack, M.; Calleja, M.; Clarke, A.; Connell, D. The prevalence and clinical significance of sonographic tendon abnormalities in asymptomatic ballet dancers: A 24-month longitudinal study. *Br. J. Sports Med.* **2013**, *47*, 89–92. [CrossRef] [PubMed]

13. Visnes, H.; Tegnander, A.; Bahr, R. Ultrasound characteristics of the patellar and quadriceps tendons among young elite athletes. *Scand. J. Med. Sci. Sports* **2015**, *25*, 205–215. [CrossRef] [PubMed]

14. Van der Worp, H.; de Poel, H.; Diercks, R.; van den Akker-Scheek, I.; Zwerver, J. Jumper's Knee or Lander's Knee? A Systematic Review of the Relation between Jump Biomechanics and Patellar Tendinopathy. *Int. J. Sports Med.* **2014**, *35*, 714–722. [CrossRef] [PubMed]

15. Reinking, M.F. Current concepts in the treatment of patellar tendinopathy. *Int. J. Sports Phys. Ther.* **2016**, *11*, 854–866. [PubMed]

16. Drakonaki, E.E.; Allen, G.M.; Wilson, D.J. Ultrasound elastography for musculoskeletal applications. *Br. J. Radiol.* **2012**, *85*, 1435–1445. [CrossRef] [PubMed]

17. Arda, K.; Ciledag, N.; Aktas, E.; Arıbas, B.K.; Köse, K. Quantitative Assessment of Normal Soft-Tissue Elasticity Using Shear-Wave Ultrasound Elastography. *Am. J. Roentgenol.* **2011**, *197*, 532–536. [CrossRef] [PubMed]

18. Zhang, Z.J.; Ng, G.Y.; Lee, W.C.; Fu, S.N. Changes in Morphological and Elastic Properties of Patellar Tendon in Athletes with Unilateral Patellar Tendinopathy and Their Relationships with Pain and Functional Disability. *PLoS ONE* **2014**, *9*, e108337. [CrossRef] [PubMed]

19. Zhang, Z.J.; Fu, S.N. Shear Elastic Modulus on Patellar Tendon Captured from Supersonic Shear Imaging: Correlation with Tangent Traction Modulus Computed from Material Testing System and Test-Retest Reliability. *PLoS ONE* **2013**, *8*, e68216. [CrossRef] [PubMed]

20. Porta, F.; Damjanov, N.; Galluccio, F.; Iagnocco, A.; Matucci-Cerinic, M. Ultrasound elastography is a reproducible and feasible tool for the evaluation of the patellar tendon in healthy subjects. *Int. J. Rheum. Dis.* **2014**, *17*, 762–766. [CrossRef] [PubMed]

21. Hsiao, M.-Y.; Chen, Y.-C.; Lin, C.-Y.; Chen, W.-S.; Wang, T.-G. Reduced Patellar Tendon Elasticity with Aging: In Vivo Assessment by Shear Wave Elastography. *Ultrasound Med. Biol.* **2015**, *41*, 2899–2905. [CrossRef] [PubMed]

22. Cook, J.L.; Khan, K.M.; Kiss, Z.S.; Coleman, B.D.; Griffiths, L. Asymptomatic hypoechoic regions on patellar tendon ultrasound: A 4-year clinical and ultrasound followup of 46 tendons. *Scand. J. Med. Sci. Sports* **2001**, *11*, 321–327. [CrossRef] [PubMed]

23. Giacchino, M.; Caresio, C.; Gorji, N.E.; Molinari, F.; Massazza, G.; Minetto, M.A. Quantitative analysis of patellar tendon size and structure in asymptomatic professional players: Sonographic study. *MLTJ* **2017**, *7*, 449–458. [CrossRef] [PubMed]

24. Pillen, S.; Tak, R.O.; Zwarts, M.J.; Lammens, M.M.Y.; Verrijp, K.N.; Arts, I.M.P.; van der Laak, J.A.; Hoogerbrugge, P.M.; van Engelen, B.G.M.; Verrips, A. Skeletal muscle ultrasound: Correlation between fibrous tissue and echo intensity. *Ultrasound Med. Biol.* **2009**, *35*, 443–446. [CrossRef] [PubMed]

25. Singh, A.P.; Singh, B. *Texture Features Extraction in Mammograms Using Non-Shannon Entropies*; Springer: Dordrecht, The Netherlands, 2010; pp. 341–351.

26. Acharya, U.R.; Krishnan, M.M.R.; Saba, L.; Molinari, F.; Guerriero, S.; Suri, J.S. Ovarian Tumor Characterization Using 3D Ultrasound. In *Ovarian Neoplasm Imaging*; Springer: Boston, MA, USA, 2013; pp. 399–412.

27. Acharya, U.R.; Faust, O.; Sree, S.V.; Molinari, F.; Suri, J.S. ThyroScreen system: High resolution ultrasound thyroid image characterization into benign and malignant classes using novel combination of texture and discrete wavelet transform. *Comput. Methods Programs Biomed.* **2012**, *107*, 233–241. [CrossRef] [PubMed]

28. Gao, S.; Peng, Y.; Guo, H.; Liu, W.; Gao, T.; Xu, Y.; Tang, X. Texture analysis and classification of ultrasound liver images. *Biomed. Mater. Eng.* **2014**, *24*, 1209–1216. [CrossRef] [PubMed]

29. Molinari, F.; Caresio, C.; Acharya, U.R.; Mookiah, M.R.K.; Minetto, M.A. Advances in Quantitative Muscle Ultrasonography Using Texture Analysis of Ultrasound Images. *Ultrasound Med. Biol.* **2015**, *41*, 2520–2532. [CrossRef] [PubMed]

30. Elias, L.J.; Bryden, M.P.; Bulman-Fleming, M.B. Footedness is a better predictor than is handedness of emotional lateralization. *Neuropsychologia* **1998**, *36*, 37–43. [CrossRef]

31. Haralick, R.M.; Shanmugam, K.; Dinstein, I. Textural Features for Image Classification. *IEEE Trans. Syst. Man Cybern.* **1973**, *6*, 610–621. [CrossRef]

32. Shao, Y.; Celenk, M. Higher-order spectra (HOS) invariants for shape recognition. *Pattern Recognit.* **2001**, *34*, 2097–2113. [CrossRef]

33. Shannon, C.E. A Mathematical Theory of Communication. *Bell Syst. Tech. J.* **1948**, *27*, 379–423. [CrossRef]

34. Rényi, A. On Measures of Entropy and Information. In Proceedings of the Fourth Berkeley Symposium on Mathematical Statistics and Probability, Berkeley, CA, USA, 14 April 1961.

35. Chen, W.; Wang, Z.; Xie, H.; Yu, W. Characterization of Surface EMG Signal Based on Fuzzy Entropy. *IEEE Trans. Neural Syst. Rehabil. Eng.* **2007**, *15*, 266–272. [CrossRef] [PubMed]

36. Kapur, J.N. Information of order α and type β. *Proc. Indian Acad. Sci.* **1968**, *68*, 65–75. [CrossRef]

37. Ghosh, M.; Chakraborty, C.; Ray, A.K. Yager's measure based fuzzy divergence for microscopic color image segmentation. In Proceedings of the 2013 Indian Conference on Medical Informatics and Telemedicine (ICMIT), Kharagpur, India, 28–30 March 2013; pp. 13–16.

38. Vajda, I. *Theory of Statistical Inference and Information*; Kluwer Academic: Dordrecht, The Netherlands, 1989; ISBN 9027727813.

39. Yin, P.-Y. Maximum entropy-based optimal threshold selection using deterministic reinforcement learning with controlled randomization. *Signal Process.* **2002**, *82*, 993–1006. [CrossRef]

40. Hu, M.-K. Visual pattern recognition by moment invariants. *IEEE Trans. Inf. Theory* **1962**, *8*, 179–187. [CrossRef]

41. Belsley, D.A.; Kuh, E.; Welsch, R.E. *Regression Diagnostics: Identifying Influential Data and Sources of Collinearity*; Wiley: Hoboken, NJ, USA, 2004; ISBN 9780471725145.

42. Hanley, J.A.; McNeil, B.J. The meaning and use of the area under a receiver operating characteristic (ROC) curve. *Radiology* **1982**, *143*, 29–36. [CrossRef] [PubMed]

43. Sharma, P.; Maffulli, N. Biology of tendon injury: Healing, modeling and remodeling. *J. Musculoskelet. Neuronal Interact.* **2006**, *6*, 181–190. [PubMed]

44. Khan, K.M.; Cook, J.L.; Bonar, F.; Harcourt, P.; Astrom, M. Histopathology of common tendinopathies. Update and implications for clinical management. *Sports Med.* **1999**, *27*, 393–408. [CrossRef] [PubMed]

45. Khan, K.M.; Maffulli, N.; Coleman, B.D.; Cook, J.L.; Taunton, J.E. Patellar tendinopathy: Some aspects of basic science and clinical management. *Br. J. Sports Med.* **1998**, *32*, 346–355. [CrossRef] [PubMed]

46. Scott, A.; Backman, L.J.; Speed, C. Tendinopathy: Update on Pathophysiology. *J. Orthop. Sports Phys. Ther.* **2015**, *45*, 833–841. [CrossRef] [PubMed]

47. Peltz, C.D.; Haladik, J.A.; Divine, G.; Siegal, D.; Van Holsbeeck, M.; Bey, M.J. ShearWave elastography: Repeatability for measurement of tendon stiffness. *Skelet. Radiol.* **2013**, *42*, 1151–1156. [CrossRef] [PubMed]

48. Aubry, S.; Nueffer, J.-P.; Tanter, M.; Becce, F.; Vidal, C.; Michel, F. Viscoelasticity in Achilles Tendonopathy: Quantitative Assessment by Using Real-time Shear-Wave Elastography. *Radiology* **2015**, *274*, 821–829. [CrossRef] [PubMed]

49. Domenichini, R.; Pialat, J.-B.; Podda, A.; Aubry, S. Ultrasound elastography in tendon pathology: State of the art. *Skelet. Radiol.* **2017**, *46*, 1643–1655. [CrossRef] [PubMed]

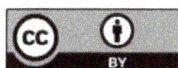

© 2018 by the authors. Licensee MDPI, Basel, Switzerland. This article is an open access article distributed under the terms and conditions of the Creative Commons Attribution (CC BY) license (http://creativecommons.org/licenses/by/4.0/).

applied sciences

MDPI

Review

Current Knowledge in Ultrasound-Based Liver Elastography of Pediatric Patients

Christoph F. Dietrich [1,*] , Roxana Sirli [2], Giovanna Ferraioli [3] , Alina Popescu [2], Ioan Sporea [2], Corina Pienar [4], Christian Kunze [5], Heike Taut [6], Simone Schrading [7], Simona Bota [8], Dagmar Schreiber-Dietrich [1] and Dong Yi [9]

[1] Medizinische Klinik 2, Caritas-Krankenhaus Bad Mergentheim, Uhlandstraße 7, 97980 Bad Mergentheim, Germany; dietrich.dagmar@googlemail.com
[2] Department of Gastroenterology and Hepatology, "Victor Babeş" University of Medicine and Pharmacy Timişoara, 300041 Timişoara, Romania; roxanasirli@gmail.com (R.S.); alinamircea.popescu@gmail.com (A.P.); isporea@umft.ro (I.S.)
[3] Ultrasound Unit, Clinical Sciences and Infectious Diseases Department, Fondazione IRCCS Policlinico San Matteo, Medical School University of Pavia, 27100 Pavia, Italy; giovanna.ferraioli@unipv.it
[4] Pediatrics Department, "Victor Babeş" University of Medicine and Pharmacy Timişoara, 300041 Timişoara, Romania; pienar.corina@umft.ro
[5] Klinik für Radiologie, Abteilung Kinderradiologie, Universitätsklinikum Halle (Saale), Martin-Luther-Universität Halle-Wittenberg, 06120 Halle, Germany; christian.kunze@uk-halle.de
[6] Klinik und Poliklinik für Kinder-und Jugendmedizin, Universitätsklinikum Carl Gustav Carus an der Technischen Universität Dresden, 01307 Dresden, Germany; Heike.Taut@uniklinikum-dresden.de
[7] Klinik für Diagnostische und Interventionelle Radiologie, University of Aachen, 52062 Aachen, Germany; sschrading@ukaachen.de
[8] Department of Gastroenterology, Hepatology, Nephrology and Endocrinology, Klinikum Klagenfurt am Wörthersee, 9020 Klagenfurt am Wörthersee, Austria; bota_simona1982@yahoo.com
[9] Department of ultrasound, Zhongshan Hospital, Fudan University, Shanghai 200433, China; drdaisydong@hotmail.com
* Correspondence: christoph.dietrich@ckbm.de; Tel.: +49-7931-58-2201

Received: 2 April 2018; Accepted: 28 May 2018; Published: 7 June 2018

Featured Application: In this review we present and discuss the published literature on the use of ultrasound-based liver elastography in children. The published data show that all the available shear wave elastography techniques are feasible and accurate for the assessment of liver fibrosis in children with diffuse liver disease due to several etiologies. For the assessment of focal liver lesions evidences are limited and no conclusion can be drawn so far.

Abstract: Studies performed using transient elastography (TE), point shear wave elastography (pSWE) and two-dimensional shear wave elastography (2D-SWE) have shown that these techniques are all feasible and accurate in children for the evaluation of liver fibrosis due to several etiologies. However, for some specific pediatric pathologies, such as biliary atresia, the evidence is still limited. As shown in adults, inflammation is a confounding factor when assessing fibrosis severity and care should be taken when interpreting the results. Due to the scarce comparative data between serological tests and elastography techniques in children, a definite conclusion regarding which is the best cannot be drawn. Neither non-invasive elastographic techniques nor laboratory scores allow determination of the presence and the degree of inflammation, necrosis, iron or copper deposits.

Keywords: ultrasound elastography; pediatric; liver fibrosis; stiffness; shear wave elastography (SWE)

1. Introduction

Ultrasound elastography is a useful non-invasive tool for the diagnosis of liver fibrosis in adults [1–7]. It plays a similar role in children, with some differences in the confounding factors and in the etiological spectrum of the liver disease; however, guidelines and recommendations have not been published yet. Preliminary data using transient elastography (TE), point shear wave elastography (pSWE) and two-dimensional shear wave elastography (2D-SWE) techniques, have shown that they are all feasible and accurate for the evaluation of liver fibrosis due to several etiologies in children [8–29]. Nonetheless, data on the use of ultrasound elastography in children younger than 6 years is still scarce. Assessment of liver stiffness is the most studied application in children. However, there are other applications of ultrasound elastography such as for the evaluation of the thyroid, renal parenchyma, bowel and testis.

Specific considerations relating to pediatric investigations include: (a) feasibility, related also to the differences in anatomy, anthropometrics, metabolic profile and psychology of each age group, the lack of cooperation to stop breathing, and so on; (b) the type of probe that should be used; (c) some differences in etiology and pathology in children; (d) cut-off values (are they the same of the adults?); (e) definition of preventable fibrosis in liver diseases.

2. Possible Indications for Shear Wave Elastography (SWE) Measurement

Currently, some chronic liver diseases can be cured or at least treated; however, follow up examinations are needed for almost all chronic liver disease for screening of complications that include liver cirrhosis, portal hypertension and malignant transformation. Close follow up is required post-liver transplantation, for autoimmune liver diseases, alpha-1 antitrypsin deficiency and cystic fibrosis [30,31]. Patients with biliary atresia, which is the most common cause of neonatal obstructive jaundice, would also benefit from non-invasive follow-up assessment after the Kasai portoenterostomy to determine the best timing for liver transplantation [29,32]. Regarding the indications, contraindications and the technique used, we refer to the published literature [33–41].

Non-alcoholic fatty liver disease (NAFLD) is the most common pediatric chronic liver diseases. It has been shown that elastography could be an excellent non-invasive tool for diagnosing and managing these patients [12,42].

Palliative surgery, such as the Fontan procedure for single ventricle hearts, may lead to longer survival, thus a higher rate of progressive hepatic failure and even hepatocellular carcinoma may be observed in these patients. Hence, the possibility to use a non-invasive tool to follow-up particular pediatric population is of paramount importance [43].

3. Elastographic Methods

According to international guidelines [1,2,4,6], ultrasound-based elastographic methods can be divided into shear wave elastography (SWE) and strain elastography (SE). The SWE techniques measure the speed of the shear waves generated in the tissues by either an external mechanical push or an ultrasound radiation force impulse (ARFI). A greater speed indicates increased tissue stiffness which is known to correlate with the dynamics and severity of fibrosis. SWE techniques can be divided into transient elastography (TE) (FibroScan®) and ARFI-based techniques. These latter are either pSWE, including Virtual Touch Quantification VTQ® from Siemens, ElastPQ® from Philips, SWM® from Hitachi, STQ® from Mindray, S-shearwave® from Samsung, QElaXto® from Esaote or 2D-SWE (first available on the Aixplorer system from SuperSonic Imagine, and later on systems from Siemens, General Electric (GE), Canon, Philips and Mindray) [4,6,44]. The speed of the shear waves is measured in meter/second (m/s); using Young's modulus it can be converted into stiffness measured in kilopascals (kPa), assuming that the tissue is purely elastic and its elastic response is linear, and that the tissue density is always 1000 kg m^{-3} [1].

3.1. Transient Elastography (TE)

Transient elastography is a non-invasive and rapid bedside method used to assess liver fibrosis by measuring liver stiffness. The technique has been described in detail in the European Federation of Societies for Ultrasound in Medicine and Biology (EFSUMB) and World Federation for Ultrasound in Medicine and Biology (WFUMB) guidelines [1,2,4,6,45] and also by others [46]. TE has been used for liver stiffness measurement (LSM) both in children and adults [1,2,47,48]. Figure 1 shows the values obtained with TE in a newborn.

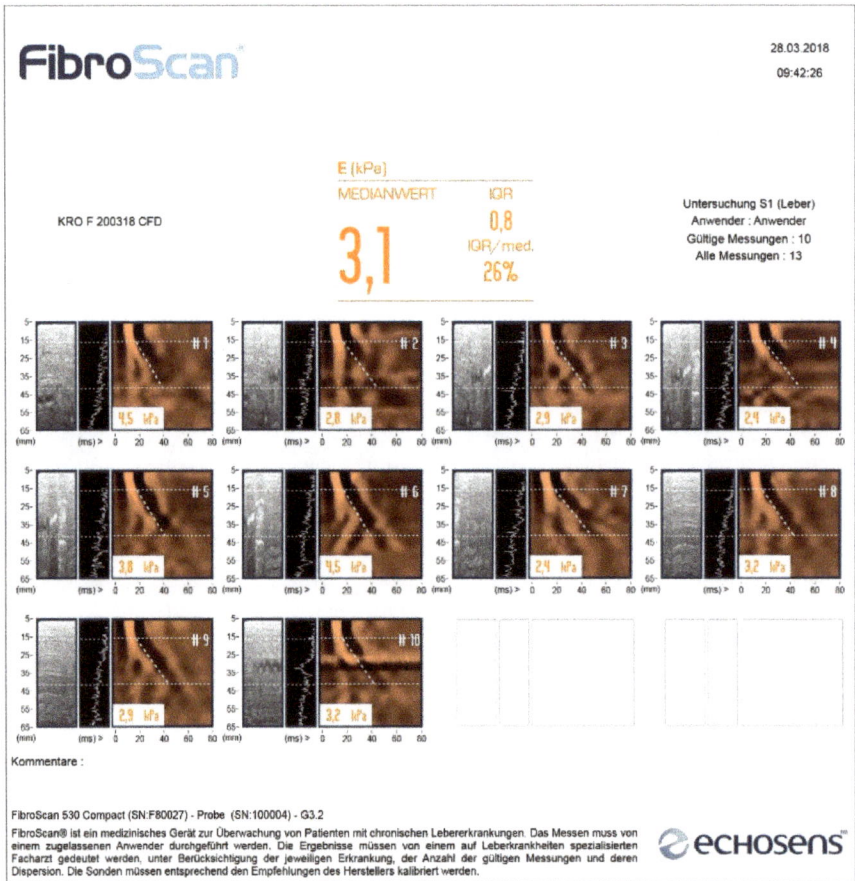

Figure 1. Transient elastography (TE) (S1 probe) in a newborn with alpha-1 antitrypsin deficiency. The individual values of 10 measurements are shown as well the median of the 10 measurements and two quality parameters, the interquartile range and the interquartile range divided by the median.

3.1.1. TE in Healthy Children

Since 2008, following the release of a new probe with a smaller diameter (S-probe 5 mm) compared to the regular probe (M-probe 7 mm), LSM using TE could be obtained in small children and infants. The feasibility of LSM in children was assessed using the S-probe (thorax perimeter < 45 cm (S1) or 45–75 cm (S2)) and the M-probe (thorax perimeter > 75 cm) according to the manufacturer's recommendations [49]. TE was technically achievable in children of all age groups. TE is feasible also in infants, but confounding factors such as the probe choice, sedation, or food intake need to be taken into account when interpreting the results. The success rate of TE decreased in children younger than 24 months even under ideal conditions. General anesthesia significantly increased LSMs in healthy children (5.4 vs. 4.2 kPa; $p < 0.01$). Probe choice equally influenced results in paired comparisons (S1 5.5 vs. S2 4.8 kPa; $p < 0.01$), as did food intake (5.9 vs. 5.4 kPa; $p = 0.015$). Inter- and intra-observer agreements were good. Normal liver stiffness was 4.5 (2.5–8.9) kPa and did not vary significantly with age or sex [50]. However, another study found that LSMs were significantly age-dependent with values of 4.40, 4.73, and 5.1 kPa in children 0–5, 6–11, and 12–18 years ($p = 0.001$) respectively (Table 1), while the interquartile range decreased with age (0.8, 0.7, and 0.6 kPa). The upper limit of normal (median plus 1.64 times standard deviation) was 5.96, 6.65, and 6.82 kPa, respectively. Girls between 11 and 18 years showed a significantly lower LSM than boys of the same age (4.7 vs. 5.6 kPa; $p < 0.005$) [48]. In younger children, the number of invalid measurements increased significantly due to movement artifacts [48], however, the measurement was reliable from the age of 6 without sedation.

Table 1. Factors that may affect measurement of liver stiffness with shear wave elastography in healthy children.

	Factor		LSM, kPa	p Value	No. of Children	Study
Transient elastography	Factor		5.5 vs. 4.8	<0.01	527	Goldschmidt et al., 2013 [1]
	Sedation (with vs. without general anesthesia)		5.4 vs. 4.2	<0.01	527	Goldschmidt et al., 2013 [1]
	Food intake (no vs. yes)		5.4 vs. 5.9	0.01	527	Goldschmidt et al., 2013 [1]
	Age (years)	0–5 vs. 6–11 vs. 12–18	4.40 vs. 4.73 vs. 5.1	0.001	240	Engelmann et al., 2012 [2]
		0–2 vs. 3–5 vs. 6–11 vs. 12–18	3.5 vs. 3.8 vs. 4.1 vs. 4.5	0.0006	173	Lewindon et al., 2016 [3]
		1–5 vs. 6–11 vs. 12–18	3.4 vs. 3.8 vs. 4.1	0.001	139	Tokuhara et al., 2016 [4]
	Gender: boys vs. girls		5.6 vs. 4.7	<0.005	240	Engelmann et al., 2012 [2]
			4.8 vs. 4.1	N.S	173	Lewindon et al., 2016 [3]
Point shear wave elastography	Probe (linear vs. convex)		SWV, m/s 1.11 vs. 1.13	0.52	109	Hanquinet et al., 2013
			1.15 vs. 1.19	N.S	60	Fontanilla et al., 2014
	Age (years)	0–1 vs. 2–5 vs. 6–10 vs. 11–18	1.05 vs. 1.00 vs. 1.12 vs. 1.12	<0.05	176	Bailey et al., 2017
		0–1 vs. 1–5 vs. 1–10 vs. 10–17	1.11 vs. 1.15 vs. 1.08 vs. 1.14	N.S	109	Hanquinet et al., 2013
		0–5 vs. 6–11 vs. 12–17	1.11 vs. 1.05 vs. 1.06	0.01	150	Matos et al., 2014
	Gender: boys vs. girls		1.08 vs. 1.08	N.S	176	Bailey et al., 2017
			1.19 vs. 1.13	0.02	132	Eiler et al., 2012
			1.11 vs. 1.14	0.3	109	Hanquinet et al., 2013
			1.07 vs. 1.08	0.47	150	Matos et al., 2014
			1.21 vs. 1.18	0.36	60	Fontanilla et al., 2014
	Left liver lobe vs. right liver lobe		1.19 vs. 1.14	0.03	132	Eiler et al., 2012
			1.21 vs. 1.07	0.000	150	Matos et al., 2014
			1.27 vs. 1.19	N.S	60	Fontanilla et al., 2014

Table 1. *Cont.*

	Factor	LSM, kPa	*p* Value	No. of Children	Study
Two-dimensional shear wave elastography	Probe (linear vs. convex)	LSM, kPa 5.96 vs. 6.94	0.006	51	Franchi-Abella et al., 2016
	Age — vs. 1–5 vs. 1–10 vs. 10–17 years	6.00 vs. 6.85 vs. 7.14 vs. 6.97	0.11	51	Franchi-Abella et al., 2016
	0–60 vs. ≥ 60 days	6.61 vs. 5.3	0.02	40	Zhou et al., 2017
	Gender: boys vs. girls	6.61 vs. 6.54	0.41	51	Franchi-Abella et al., 2016
		5.4 vs. 5.6	0.63	40	Zhou et al., 2017

Explanations: LSM: liver stiffness measurement; kPa: kilopascal, SWV: shear wave velocity; N.S non-significant; m/s: meter per second.

As shown in Table 1, in a series of non-sedated control group of children LSM also increased with age; 0–2 years (3.5 ± 0.5 kPa), 3–5 years (3.8 ± 0.3 kPa) and 6–11 years (4.1 ± 0.2 kPa), with healthy older children 12–18 years having values similar to adults (4.5 ± 0.2 kPa). LSM did not vary significantly with gender (female, 4.5 ± 0.2 vs. male, 4.8 ± 0.2 kPa). Children with non-hepatic illnesses had higher LSM (5.2 ± 0.2 kPa) compared to healthy children (4.1 ± 0.1 kPa) [51].

Another study has confirmed that LSM increased with age: it was 3.4 kPa (2.3–4.6 kPa) at ages 1–5 years; 3.8 (2.5–6.1) kPa at ages 6–11; and 4.1 (3.3–7.9) kPa at ages 12–18 ($p = 0.001$). The M-probe was suitable in a wide age range of children from age 1 year onwards. In children without evidence of liver disease, LSM showed an age-dependent increase [23].

Still, when using the M probe in children with a thoracic perimeter below 45 cm, one should consider the "underestimation" phenomenon. It has been shown that LSM decreased with probe size (S1 < S2 < M) and caution is needed when interpreting the results [52].

3.1.2. TE in Non-Alcoholic Fatty Liver Disease (NAFLD)

In children with NAFLD (age range from 5.5 to 11.3 years), the combination of pediatric NAFLD fibrosis index (PNFI) and TE were used to assess the presence of clinically significant liver fibrosis. Both PNFI and TE values were significantly higher in children with significant fibrosis [53]. The combined use of PNFI and TE predicted the presence or absence of clinically significant fibrosis in 98% of children with NAFLD. This could help to identify children who should undergo liver biopsy because the confirmation of advanced fibrosis would lead to closer follow up and screening for cirrhosis-related complications.

In a series of 52 biopsy-proven pediatric non-alcoholic steatohepatitis (NASH), the following cutoffs for staging liver fibrosis were found: 5–7 kPa for F1 (area under the receiver-operating characteristic (AUROC) curve, 97.7%), 7–9 kPa for F2 (AUROC, 99.2%), >9 kPa for F3 (AUROC, 100%) [42].

3.1.3. Correlation with Fibrosis Stage and Different Etiologies

LSM using TE in pediatric patients with chronic liver disease correlated significantly with both fibrosis area fraction [54] and Ishak scores, the correlation appearing better with the latter (r = 0.839 vs. 0.879, $p < 0.0001$ for both). LSM discriminated individual stages of fibrosis with high performance. Sensitivity ranged from 81.4% to 100% and specificity ranged from 75.0 to 97.2%. However, LSMs for the same stage of fibrosis varied according to different etiologies. For example, for F3 Ishak stage, higher values were obtained in children with autoimmune hepatitis (16.15 ± 7.23 kPa) compared to those with Wilson's disease (8.30 ± 0.84 kPa) and hepatitis C virus (HCV) hepatitis (7.43 ± 1.73 kPa).

Multiple regression analysis revealed that Ishak fibrosis stage was the only independent variable associated with higher LSM ($p < 0.0001$) [17].

In a study that prospectively included 116 consecutive children with chronic liver diseases, de Ledinghen et al. reported that the AUROCs for the diagnosis of cirrhosis were 0.88, 0.73, and 0.73 for FibroScan, Fibrotest, and Aspartateaminotransferase-to-Platelet Ratio Index (APRI), respectively. The FibroScan equipped with the specific smaller diameter probe (S-probe 5 mm) could become a useful tool for the management of chronic liver diseases in children [49].

In a pediatric cohort, TE findings were compared with the ability of serum hyaluronic acid (HA) and human cartilage glycoprotein-39 (YKL-40) values in predicting advanced hepatic fibrosis [55]. For the prediction of advanced fibrosis, TE showed an AUROC significantly higher (0.83) than HA (0.72) or YKL-40 (0.52). The optimal TE cut-off value for predicting F3–F4 fibrosis was 8.6 kPa. The combination of TE and HA was not better than TE alone for predicting advanced fibrosis [56].

Studies in adults have shown that inflammation increases liver stiffness, leading to an overestimation of fibrosis. The influence of inflammation to LSMs in children/young adults has been investigated as well. In patients with fibrosis stages F0–F2, the proportion of those with LSM > 8.6 kPa increased with increasing alanine aminotransferase (ALT). In patients with F3–F4, there was no association between ALT and LSM. A weak correlation between a change in ALT and LSM was observed in patients with no/minimal fibrosis and inflammatory liver diseases (r = 0.33). In children with no/minimal hepatic fibrosis and inflammatory liver disease, high ALT values were associated with LSM in the range typical for advanced fibrosis. However, with more advanced fibrosis, inflammation did not appear to contribute to LSM. Caution must be taken when interpreting LSM for assessing fibrosis severity in the setting of inflammation [11].

TE may be useful in follow-up of children following Fontan surgery. The technique is feasible and it has been reported that pediatric Fontan patients have markedly elevated LSMs (18.6 versus 4.7 kPa) [18]. There was no association between TE values and patient age, time since Fontan surgery, or median Fontan circuit pressure. [18].

The liver stiffness score of biliary atresia patients was significantly higher than that of normal controls (27.37 ± 22.48 and 4.69 ± 1.03 kPa; $p < 0.001$). The sensitivity (and specificity) of TE (using a cut-off value of 12.7 kPa) and APRI (using a cut-off value of 1.92) in predicting esophageal/gastric varices were 84% (77%) and 84% (83%), respectively [57].

3.2. Point SWE (pSWE)

The technique has been described in detail in the EFSUMB and WFUMB guidelines [1,2,4,6].

Trout et al. reported that pSWE and magnetic resonance elastography (MRE) values correlated well in patients with a body mass index (BMI) of less than 30 kg/m² and minimal US data dispersion; increasing US data dispersion was directly related to a higher BMI [27]. In another study, SWVs differed between normal-weight and obese children (1.08 ± 0.14 versus 1.44 ± 0.39 m/s; $p < 0.001$), but not by gender. Multivariate linear regression demonstrated that the shear wave velocities (SWV)s were primarily associated with age in normal-weight children ($p < 0.05$) and with BMI in obese children ($p < 0.001$). In the obese group, mean SWV was significantly higher in children with abnormal echogenic livers than in those with livers of normal appearance (1.53 ± 0.38 vs. 1.17 ± 0.27), $p < 0.05$. The difference was not significant in the normal-weight group [58].

In the study of Eiler et al., which included 132 patients 0–17 years, the mean value of SWV was 1.16 (0.14) m/s. Neither age ($p = 0.533$) nor depth of measurement ($p = 0.066$) had a significant influence on SWV, whereas a significant effect of gender was found, with lower values in females ($n = 71$, $p = 0.025$); however, there was no significant interaction between age groups (before or after puberty) and gender ($p = 0.276$). There was an inter-lobar difference with lower values in the right liver lobe compared to the left (1.14 ± 0.22 m/s vs. 1.19 ± 0.28 m/s, $p = 0.036$) and with a significantly lower variance in the right lobe ($p < 0.001$). Consistent values were measured by different examiners ($p = 0.108$); however, the inter-examiner variance deviated significantly ($p < 0.001$) [59].

SWV measurement was feasible in children at any age with acceptable reliability. The depth of measurements in the liver seemed to have no influence on the results. There was no statistical difference between measurements taken at different ages, with a mean SWV of 1.12 m/s (range: 0.73 to 1.45 m/s) [60].

In another study, mean SWV in the right liver lobe was 1.07 ± 0.10 m/s. No significant differences were found according to sex or among different probe locations [61]. SWVs were, however, significantly higher in the left liver lobe in comparison to the right lobe (1.07 ± 0.10 m/s, right; 1.21 ± 0.16 m/s, left). The depth of measurements also influenced the SWV values, being slightly lower at deeper locations. Regarding the age, significant differences were found for children <6 years old compared with other age groups. SWV seems to be influenced by age, depth, and measurement location. A mean SWV of 1.07 ± 0.10 m/s for a healthy pediatric population with the possibility of reaching 1.12 m/s in the case of younger children was found. SWV values were more consistently obtained when assessing the right liver lobe and at depths lower than 5 to 6 cm [61].

pSWE and 2D-SWE values were able to detect high-grade histopathological fibrosis and had high success rates when distinguishing high-grade from low-grade fibrosis. In a series of 75 children, SWV cut offs were 1.67 m/s for pSWE and 1.56 m/s for 2D-SWE in detecting fibrosis or inflammation and 2.09 m/s for pSWE and 2.17 m/s for 2D-SWE in discriminating children with low and high histological liver fibrosis scores. However, both techniques had limited success rates when differentiating low-grade fibrosis from normal liver tissue [14]. In another prospective study, pSWE was feasible in children using both the convex and the linear transducers. Mean SWV measured in the right lobe was 1.19 ± 0.04 m/s with the convex transducer and 1.15 ± 0.04 m/s with the linear transducer. Age had a small effect on the measurements. BMI and gender had no significant effects on SWV, whereas site of measurement had a significant effect, with lower SWV values in the right hepatic lobe. The authors suggested that the SWV values obtained in the right lobe may be used as reference values for normal liver stiffness in children [62].

Another prospective study in 235 healthy children (6–17 years) showed also a significant difference between the values of right and left liver lobe and a small influence of age and gender with lower values in older children and significant lower values in females after puberty. It was suggested that best point of examination is the right lobe in the interaxillar line with transverse transducer direction [62].

3.2.1. Liver Fibrosis

Quantification of liver fibrosis correlates with the histological fibrosis stage in children with chronic liver disease [63]. The accuracy of pSWE in determining the extent of liver fibrosis in pediatric patients with short bowel syndrome has been evaluated. The AUROCs to differentiate moderate/severe liver fibrosis from mild disease were 0.83 and 0.86 for the median and mean SWV, respectively [10].

In children without inflammation, SWV was higher when fibrosis was present compared to the absence of fibrosis (average SWV 1.8 vs. 1.4 m/s). A SWV cut-off of 1.7 m/s had 100% positive predictive value and 24% negative predictive value for detecting liver fibrosis or inflammation [15].

Fibrosis related to several causes can be diagnosed in children and adolescents' liver grafts. In a small series (30 subjects), the AUROCs for SWV, APRI, and AST/ALT (aspartate aminotransferase/alanine aminotransferase) ratio index for significant fibrosis were 0.76, 0.74, and 0.69, respectively. Through multivariate logistic regression analysis, the only independent predictor of significant fibrosis was SWV. SWV assessment may serve as a potential method for assessing significant fibrosis in pediatric patients with liver transplants, particularly in combination with AST/ALT ratio [64].

Graft fibrosis is a common finding from biopsies after pediatric liver transplantation. LSMs had good accuracy for diagnosing graft fibrosis after pediatric living donor liver transplantation. SWVs significantly increased with increased portal and pericellular fibrosis grades [65]. For the diagnosis of significant fibrosis, the AUROCs were 0.760 and 0.849 for the midline and intercostal values, respectively, and the optimal cut-off values were 1.30 and 1.39 m/s for midline and intercostal values. The pericellular pattern of fibrosis was frequently observed in this setting, and moderate pericellular fibrosis was detectable by SWV [65].

3.2.2. Values in Obesity

The mean pSWE value was 1.13 (0.20) m/s for obese children and 1.02 (0.11) m/s for children in the control group, whereas other authors did not find any statistically significant influence of the BMI on pSWE values [66–69]. SWV showed excellent correlation with AST/ALT ratios in obese children and may be used as a non-invasive tool to detect NAFLD and associated hepatic changes, especially in pediatric patients, for whom liver biopsy is not always feasible [9].

3.2.3. Liver Disease Associated with Cystic Fibrosis (CFLD)

Liver disease associated with cystic fibrosis (CFLD) is the second cause of mortality in these patients [31,70]. Comparing the SWV values of CFLD with those of a control healthy group, values in the right lobe were higher in patients with CFLD. A SWV cut-off value to detect CFLD of 1.27 m/s with a sensitivity of 56.5% and a specificity of 90.5% has been reported. Cystic fibrosis patients were found to have higher SWV spleen values than the control group, without any clinical consequence. A study that enrolled children with liver disease, found that a value of 1.16 m/s ($\pm$0.14 m/s) allows a differentiation of healthy versus pathological liver tissue [30].

3.3. Two-Dimensional Shear Wave Elastography (2D-SWE)

The technique has been described in detail in the EFSUMB and WFUMB guidelines [1,2,4,6]. A 2D-SWE techinique is exemplified in Figure 2.

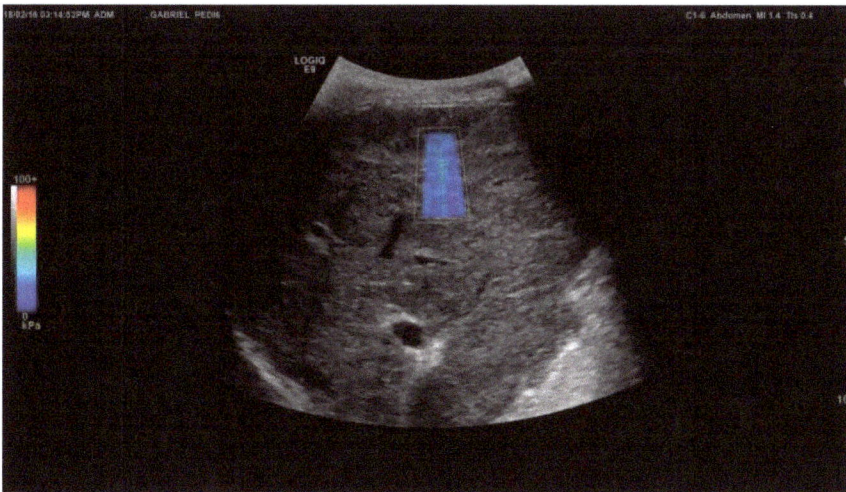

Figure 2. Two-dimensional shear wave elastography (2D-SWE) in a 10 years old boy with cystic fibrosis associated liver disease. The median of liver stiffness measurements using the convex probe was 4.47 kPa, IQR = 1.13. Point SWE results were 1.47 m/s (convex probe).

A recent meta-analysis analyzed 12 studies on 550 patients to assess the diagnostic performance of 2D-SWE for determining the severity of liver fibrosis in children and adolescents. The summary sensitivity was 81% (95% CI: 71–88) and the specificity was 91% (95% CI: 83–96) for the prediction of significant liver fibrosis. Subgroup analysis revealed that 2D-SWE had an excellent diagnostic performance according to each degree of liver fibrosis. 2D-SWE had a higher sensitivity ($p < 0.01$) and specificity ($p < 0.01$) than VTQ® [71]. In this meta-analysis, the number of LSMs performed was a significant factor influencing study heterogeneity.

3.3.1. Technical Success Rates of Liver Stiffness Estimates

Five studies on healthy subjects and/or patients with chronic liver diseases have reported results on the technical success rate of 2D-SWE in pediatric patients. In two studies on, respectively, 96 and 88 subjects, no technical failure was observed [72,73]. In another study on NASH pediatric patients, 2D-SWE was feasible in 68/69 (99%) of them [12]. In a large series, the success rates of LSMs in the study group and the control group were 96.4% (244/253) and 100% (40/40), respectively [73]. The main reasons for failure were crying and body movements. No technical failure was observed in a free-breathing status [72]. A more recent study evaluated the stability index (SI) of 2D-SWE acquisitions as a quality indicator of measurements [74]. Using an SI < 90% as an indicator of unreliable measurement, failure to obtain reliable 2D-SWE measurements was observed in five of 29 patients (17%) in the free-breathing group and in two of 29 patients (7%) in the breath-holding group. Comparison of the mean elasticity value revealed no significant difference between free breathing and breath-holding (6.31 ± 3.98 kPa vs. 6.47 ± 4.09 kPa, $p = 0.354$, $n = 29$) [74].

Hepatic 2D-SWE performed with free breathing yielded results similar to the breath-hold condition. With a substantially lower time requirement, which could be further reduced by lowering the number of acquisitions, it was concluded that the free-breathing technique may be suitable for infants and less cooperative children not capable of breath-holding [13].

3.3.2. Reproducibility and Variability of Liver Stiffness Estimates

The intra-operator reproducibility of LSMs was found to be excellent, comparing the average of 3, 5 or 7 measurements to the average of 15 considered as the reference, with intraclass correlation coefficient (ICC) of 0.944 (95% CI: 0.899–0.972), 0.958 (95% CI: 0.923–0.978) and 0.969 (95% CI: 0.945–0.982), respectively, in free-breathing status. Results were very similar in the group of patients studied with breath-hold: ICC = 0.937 (95% CI: 0.887–0.978), ICC = 0.938 (95% CI: 0.876–0.981), and ICC = 0.941 (95% CI: 0.878–0.983) for the average of 3, 5 and 7 measurements, respectively [74]. An excellent correlation of repeated measurements made by each of three operators was also reported in another study, with intra-operator ICCs ranging from 0.93 to 0.96 [73]. This study also investigated inter-observer agreement in 39 randomly selected children (9 controls, 16 patients without biliary atresia (BA) and 14 with BA. Very good reproducibility was found among the three operators (ICC = 0.98; 95% CI: 0.96–0.99), and the Bland–Altman analysis also showed that the interobserver agreements within each pair of operators were good [73].

Another study on NASH patients with various stages of liver fibrosis (F0: $n = 5$; F1: $n = 16$; F2–3: $n = 14$) showed that the inter-observer agreement between two operators was excellent, as indicated by an ICC for absolute agreement of 0.95 (95% CI: 0.90, 0.97) [12]. Using the SI as an indicator of unreliable measurements, it has been found that an intra-operator ICC of 0.87 (95% CI, 0.74 to 0.94) in the free-breathing group increased to 0.99 (95% CI, 0.97 to 0.99) when the SI was used. Similarly, the ICC of 0.95 (95% CI, 0.90 to 0.98) in the breath-holding group increased to 0.99 (95% CI, 0.99 to 0.99) when the SI was used [74].

3.3.3. Liver Stiffness Estimates in Healthy Controls

Liver stiffness estimates in healthy subjects have been assessed in several studies, and most information comes from the control group of case-control studies. The mean 2D-SWE value was 5.5 ± 1.3 kPa in free-breathing status and 5.5 ± 1.1 kPa, with a range of 3.7–7.7 kPa [73]. The breathing method does not seem to have an impact on 2D-SWE values and their variability [72,73]. The gender seems not to significantly affect 2D-SWE values [73], with average values of 5.4 ± 1.1 kPa in males versus 5.6 ± 1.1 kPa in females ($p = 0.637$) [73]. LSMs were found to correlate with children's age (r = 0.429, p = 0.006), and to be significantly higher (6.1 ± 1.1 kPa) in babies older than 60 days (n = 10) than in babies of 60 days or below (5.3 ± 1.0 kPa) (n = 30) (p = 0.026) [73]. However, another study didn't find any significant difference between different age groups (p = 0.11) [25] and only a trend to an increase of LSMs with age was found when using the linear transducer (p = 0.05). Technical factors may also affect LSMs, including the transducer used: a significant difference was found for mean elasticity between the linear and convex transducers: 5.96 kPa ± 1.31 and 6.94 kPa ± 1.42, respectively (p = 0.006) [25].

3.3.4. Number of Measurements Needed

2D-SWE enables evaluation of the velocity of several shear wave fronts in real-time. There are no specific manufacturer recommendations on how many measurements are sufficient to obtain reliable results. In addition, repeating procedures to obtain 10 measurements is challenging in children. The mean LSMs obtained with three, five and seven acquisitions demonstrated almost perfect agreement with the reference obtained with 15 acquisitions in both free-breathing and breath-holding status. Three acquisitions can be enough for hepatic LSMs in children older than 6 years regardless of breathing status or hepatic pathology. More acquisitions are recommended for children under the age of 5 years during free breathing [72]. To reach an acceptable liver stiffness error range below 5%, the use of the SI to identify unreliable measurements was found to reduce the number of acquisitions required from 8 to 5 in the free-breathing group, and from 6 to 2 in the breath-hold group [74].

3.3.5. Pediatric Patients with NAFLD

2D-SWE is an accurate and reproducible non-invasive technique that efficiently depicts the presence of significant liver fibrosis and, less accurately, mild liver fibrosis in pediatric patients with NAFLD. 2D-SWE showed a very high correlation with liver fibrosis (p < 0.001) at univariate and multivariate analyses. The AUROCs for the association of any and significant fibrosis were 0.92 and 0.97, respectively [12].

3.3.6. Liver Fibrosis in Biliary Atresia (BA) Patients

The availability of an effective non-invasive tool for monitoring liver fibrosis in children with BA is important, but evidence is limited. 2D-SWE is a more promising tool to assess liver fibrosis than APRI and fibrosis-4 (FIB-4) in children with BA after the Kasai procedure. The AUROCs of 2D-SWE, APRI and their combination were 0.79, 0.65 and 0.78 for significant fibrosis; 0.81, 0.64 and 0.76 for advanced fibrosis; and 0.82, 0.56 and 0.84 for cirrhosis, respectively [19].

LSM was found to be higher in patients with BA as compared to controls: 12.6 kPa (10.6–18.8) versus 9.6 kPa (7.5–11.7) (p < 0.001), without any difference between gender (p = 0.071) [73]. The difference in LSMs between BA patients and controls also applied to the two age groups using the 60-day age cutoff (p < 0.001 below age cutoff and p = 0.002 above age cutoff). Using a cutoff value ≥10.2 kPa, the sensitivity, specificity, positive predictive value and negative predictive value for the diagnosis of BA were 81.4%, 66.7%, 76.0%, and 73.5%, respectively. Using the same cutoff value, the sensitivity of the test improved to 92.5% in the >60 days old age group (n = 60), whereas it decreased to 68.2% in younger babies (n = 53). In these patients, age, direct and indirect bilirubin levels significantly correlated with LSM (all p < 0.001), whereas both ALT and AST levels did not correlate (both p > 0.05) [73]. In 12 patients after the Kasai intervention (M:F = 3:9, mean age 9.3 ± 4.4 years, age range 3–18 years old), without clinical evidence of acute illness including cholangitis, and no incidental mass or cystic lesion in the liver, the mean value from fifteen LSMs was 8.0 ± 2.2 kPa.

3.3.7. Intrahepatic Portal Hypertension

LSM has been significantly correlated with hepatic venous-pressure gradient (HVPG). The AUROC for predicting clinically significant portal hypertension was 0.914, and the best cut-off value of 18.4 kPa showed sensitivity of 87.5% and specificity of 84.0%. 2D-SWE had excellent diagnostic performance for predicting clinically significant portal hypertension in children with suspected liver diseases. It has been suggested that a coefficient of variation (CV) ≤ 0.2 may possibly be used as a reliability criterion in 2D-SWE measurement [16].

3.3.8. Focal Liver Lesions

Evidences are limited and no conclusion can be drawn. In a case-control study on 20 patients with hepatic tumors, stiffness estimates of malignant tumors by two operators were found to be significantly higher ($p = 0.02$) than that of hepatic hemangiomas: 47 kPa and 58 kPa for malignant lesions versus 22 kPa and 24 kPa, respectively, for both operators. The AUROC of SWE for differentiating hepatic hemangiomas from malignant hepatic tumors was 0.77 with a sensitivity of 72.7% and a specificity of 66.7%, using a cutoff value of 23.62 kPa. IContrast-enhanced ultrasound (CEUS) is used for the improved detection and characterization of focal liver lesions [75–81]. CEUS does not influence the measurement of liver stiffness [82].

3.4. Strain Imaging (Real-Time Elastography (RTE))

Real-time elastography (RTE) has been used mainly for the evaluation of the pancreas [83–86], the thyroid [87–94], the prostate [95], the breast [5,96] but also for the liver [1,2,7,97]. Published evidence in children is scarce and contradictory [98–100].

4. Comparison of TE, pSWE and 2D-SWE

Using TE as a reference method, sensitivity of pSWE was 71.42% for detecting F1 fibrosis, 77.77% for F2, 62.5% for F3, and 71.42% for F4. Sensitivity of 2D-SWE was 92.85% for detecting F1, 83.33% for F2, 87.5 % for F3, and 85.71 % for F4. Significant correlation was found between TE and 2D-SWE overall (Kappa correlation factor = 0.843, $p = 0.001$). Analyzing the subgroup with success rate (SR) = 60–70%, no significant correlation between TE and pSWE was found (Kappa correlation factor = 0.172, $p = 0.452$). Assessing the subgroup with SR > 70%, a significant correlation between TE and pSWE was found (Kappa correlation factor = 0.761, $p = 0.001$). Overall, 2D-SWE correlated with TE better than pSWE [24].

5. What Is the Benefit of SWE in Children?

Invasive methods for the evaluation of the severity of liver diseases in children are more difficult to perform. Sedation is sometimes necessary, the parents and the children are afraid of the procedure and its complications, especially if repeated procedures are needed for follow-up. Thus, in this population the need for non-invasive modalities of evaluation is of great interest. The main advantages of ARFI-based elastography techniques are that they are rapid, repeatable when necessary, not expensive and available in high-end ultrasound machines. Moreover, they are painless, take less than 5 min and little cooperation is needed from the child. In infants, the procedures may take longer time since cooperation from the patient is more difficult, and may require parent support. On the other hand, liver biopsy, which is the reference standard for fibrosis staging, has several limitations, including bleeding and possible surgery, the possible need for sedation, pain, fear and others, so it is not always feasible in the follow-up of patients with chronic parenchymal liver diseases [36,37,40,69].

5.1. What Is Best in Children: TE, pSWE or 2D-SWE and Why?

As for the adult population, maybe it is too early to answer this question. Each method has its strong points, including feasibility, reproducibility, acceptable number of false positive or negative results. TE is quick to perform and very little cooperation is needed. It is also the most studied technique since it was the first available on the market. On the other hand, the cost of the machine and the additional cost for probe calibration in a system that is not embedded in an ultrasound machine should be considered. However, it is a unique device that has also the advantage of steatosis assessment by controlled attenuation parameter (CAP). pSWE and 2D-SWE techniques are available on conventional high-end ultrasound machines and have the advantage of good feasibility. Moreover, these techniques are accurate in staging liver fibrosis. Future comparative, prospective studies are necessary for the definitive answer to this question.

5.2. Scores in Fatty Liver Disease and Fibrosis: Are They Better than SWE?

Another alternative for the non-invasive assessment of liver fibrosis are the serologic tests such as FibroTest, APRI, Forns Index, Fib-4, NAFLD test, PNFI, pediatric NAFLD fibrosis score (PNFS), and so on. FibroTest-ActiTest has been validated in children with chronic hepatitis C [101,102]. Only a few studies have been published regarding the comparative value of ultrasound-based elastographic techniques and serologic tests. In a pilot study, it was found that, for the diagnosis of cirrhosis, the AUROCs for TE, FibroTest, and APRI were 0.88, 0.73, and 0.73, respectively [49]. In an Egyptian cohort, the AUROCs of TE and APRI score for discriminating significant fibrosis (F2, Metavir score) were 0.883 and 0.746, while the correlations with liver biopsy were 0.58 and 0.53, respectively [21].

The advantages of serological tests are that they do not require any specialized equipment, however patented tests are expensive and not readily available. FibroTest-ActiTest, even though expensive, has the advantage of giving information regarding the severity of inflammation.

Considering the scarce comparative data between serology and elastography tests in children, a definite conclusion regarding which one is the best cannot be drawn.

6. Limits of Liver Elastography

Neither non-invasive elastographic techniques nor laboratory scores allow a determination of the presence and the degree of inflammation, necrosis, fat deposits (micro- or macro-vesicular, mixed) and iron or copper deposits. Elastography does not replace biopsy and histological evaluation in autoimmune hepatitis including treatment control and some other forms of acute and chronic liver disease before and after transplantation. Elastographic techniques cannot discriminate between contiguous stages of fibrosis (F0 vs.F1; F1 vs. F2). Quality parameters are of importance [103].

Some prognostically important markers such as portal inflammation and the exact degree of fibrosis are best determined by liver biopsy [28,104]. It seems clear that SWE cannot replace all information shown in the complex published scores for adult and pediatric patients (e.g., Desmet (CHC), METAVIR and Ishak (CHC, CHB)) to evaluate the necro-inflammatory activity (grading) and stage of fibrosis. The Semiquantitaive Scoring System (SSS) of Chevallier was developed to quantify fibrosis irrespective of the underlying disease. In a series of 430 obese children the association and prognosis of portal inflammation, metabolic syndrome and fibrosis was shown only with histology [28]. This information cannot be obtained with non-invasive measurements.

7. Conclusions

SWE techniques have increasingly been used in children with several etiologies of diffuse liver disease. Each technique has its strong points, including feasibility, reproducibility, acceptable number of false positive or negative results. TE is quick to perform and very little cooperation is needed. It is also the most studied method since it was the first available on the market. Point SWE and 2D-SWE techniques are available on conventional high-end ultrasound machines and have the advantage of allowing the morphological assessment of the liver in B-mode as well.

Studies have shown that all SWE techniques are feasible in children at any age with acceptable reliability. LSMs values seem age-dependent, with children of age 12 or more having values similar to adults. The majority of studies have shown that girls have significantly lower LSMs than boys of the same age; however some studies did not confirm this finding. SWE is feasible also in babies but confounding factors such as the probe choice, sedation, or food intake need to be taken into account when interpreting the results.

As reported in adults, LSMs obtained in the right liver lobe are lower than those obtained in the left lobe, and measurements should be performed in the right lobe whenever possible. The majority of studies have shown that LSMs are not influenced by the BMI.

The intra-operator reproducibility of LSMs by 2D-SWE was found to be excellent and the breathing does not seem to affect the results. Three 2D-SWE acquisitions can be enough for hepatic LSMs in children older than 6 years old regardless of breathing status or hepatic pathology. More acquisitions seem needed for children under the age of five during free breathing.

Ultrasound elastography is a reliable non-invasive method to monitor liver fibrosis in pediatric patients. However, for some pathologies, such as biliary atresia, the evidence is still limited. As shown in adults, inflammation is a confounding factor when assessing fibrosis severity and care should be taken when interpreting the results. Elastographic techniques cannot discriminate between contiguous stages of fibrosis (F0 vs. F1; F1 vs. F2). Moreover, as reported in adults, LSMs for the same stage of fibrosis vary according to different etiologies of liver disease and different values are obtained with different ultrasound systems.

Due to the scarce comparative data between serology and elastography techniques in children, a definite conclusion regarding which is the best cannot be drawn. Neither non-invasive elastographic techniques nor laboratory scores allow a determination of the presence and the degree of inflammation, necrosis, iron or copper deposits.

Acknowledgments: We acknowledge the discussion with Gerhard Alzen, Giessen, Germany. We acknowledge the support of the Bad Mergentheimer Leberzentrum e.V.

Conflicts of Interest: Christoph F Dietrich, speaker for: Hitachi Medical Systems, Siemens Healthineers, Mindray Medical Systems, Supersonic, GE, Bracco, Pentax, Olympus, Fuji, Boston Scientific, AbbVie, Falk, Novartis. Giovanna Ferraioli: Philips Healthcare, Canon Medical Systems, Hitachi Medical Systems, Mindray Medical Systems. Roxana Sirli: I have received financial support (congress travel grant or speaker fees) from Philips, Abbvie, Zentiva. Alina Popescu: I have received financial support (congress travel grants, speaker fees) from: Philips, General Electric, Abbvie, AstraZeneca, Zentiva. Ioan Sporea: I have received financial support (congress travel grant or speaker fees) from Philips, Siemens, General Electric, Abbvie, Zentiva, Bristol Meyers Squibb. Corina Pienar and Christian Kunze declare no conflict of interest.

References

1. Dietrich, C.F.; Bamber, J.; Berzigotti, A.; Bota, S.; Cantisani, V.; Castera, L.; Cosgrove, D.; Ferraioli, G.; Friedrich-Rust, M.; Gilja, O.H.; et al. EFSUMB guidelines and recommendations on the clinical use of liver ultrasound elastography, update 2017 (long version). *Ultraschall Med.* **2017**, *38*, e16–e47. [CrossRef] [PubMed]
2. Dietrich, C.F.; Bamber, J.; Berzigotti, A.; Bota, S.; Cantisani, V.; Castera, L.; Cosgrove, D.; Ferraioli, G.; Friedrich-Rust, M.; Gilja, O.H.; et al. EFSUMB guidelines and recommendations on the clinical use of liver ultrasound elastography, update 2017 (short version). *Ultraschall Med.* **2017**, *38*, 377–394. [CrossRef] [PubMed]
3. Dong, Y.; Sirli, R.; Ferraioli, G.; Sporea, I.; Chiorean, L.; Cui, X.; Fan, M.; Wang, W.P.; Gilja, O.H.; Sidhu, P.S.; et al. Shear wave elastography of the liver—Review on normal values. *Z. Gastroenterol.* **2017**, *55*, 153–166. [CrossRef] [PubMed]
4. Bamber, J.; Cosgrove, D.; Dietrich, C.F.; Fromageau, J.; Bojunga, J.; Calliada, F.; Cantisani, V.; Correas, J.M.; D'Onofrio, M.; Drakonaki, E.E.; et al. Efsumb guidelines and recommendations on the clinical use of ultrasound elastography. Part 1: Basic principles and technology. *Ultraschall Med.* **2013**, *34*, 169–184. [CrossRef] [PubMed]
5. Cosgrove, D.; Piscaglia, F.; Bamber, J.; Bojunga, J.; Correas, J.M.; Gilja, O.H.; Klauser, A.S.; Sporea, I.; Calliada, F.; Cantisani, V.; et al. Efsumb guidelines and recommendations on the clinical use of ultrasound elastography. Part 2: Clinical applications. *Ultraschall Med.* **2013**, *34*, 238–253. [PubMed]
6. Shiina, T.; Nightingale, K.R.; Palmeri, M.L.; Hall, T.J.; Bamber, J.C.; Barr, R.G.; Castera, L.; Choi, B.I.; Chou, Y.H.; Cosgrove, D.; et al. Wfumb guidelines and recommendations for clinical use of ultrasound elastography: Part 1: Basic principles and terminology. *Ultrasound Med. Biol.* **2015**, *41*, 1126–1147. [CrossRef] [PubMed]

7. Ferraioli, G.; Filice, C.; Castera, L.; Choi, B.I.; Sporea, I.; Wilson, S.R.; Cosgrove, D.; Dietrich, C.F.; Amy, D.; Bamber, J.C.; et al. Wfumb guidelines and recommendations for clinical use of ultrasound elastography: Part 3: Liver. *Ultrasound Med. Biol.* **2015**, *41*, 1161–1179. [CrossRef] [PubMed]

8. Ferraioli, G.; Calcaterra, V.; Lissandrin, R.; Guazzotti, M.; Maiocchi, L.; Tinelli, C.; De Silvestri, A.; Regalbuto, C.; Pelizzo, G.; Larizza, D.; et al. Noninvasive assessment of liver steatosis in children: The clinical value of controlled attenuation parameter. *BMC Gastroenterol.* **2017**, *17*, 61. [CrossRef] [PubMed]

9. Kamble, R.; Sodhi, K.S.; Thapa, B.R.; Saxena, A.K.; Bhatia, A.; Dayal, D.; Khandelwal, N. Liver acoustic radiation force impulse (ARFI) in childhood obesity: Comparison and correlation with biochemical markers. *J. Ultrasound* **2017**, *20*, 33–42. [CrossRef] [PubMed]

10. Lodwick, D.; Dienhart, M.; Cooper, J.N.; Fung, B.; Lopez, J.; Smith, S.; Warren, P.; Balint, J.; Minneci, P.C. A pilot study of ultrasound elastography as a non-invasive method to monitor liver disease in children with short bowel syndrome. *J. Pediatr. Surg.* **2017**, *52*, 962–965. [CrossRef] [PubMed]

11. Raizner, A.; Shillingford, N.; Mitchell, P.D.; Harney, S.; Raza, R.; Serino, J.; Jonas, M.M.; Lee, C.K. Hepatic inflammation may influence liver stiffness measurements by transient elastography in children and young adults. *J. Pediatr. Gastroenterol. Nutr.* **2017**, *64*, 512–517. [CrossRef] [PubMed]

12. Garcovich, M.; Veraldi, S.; Di Stasio, E.; Zocco, M.A.; Monti, L.; Toma, P.; Pompili, M.; Gasbarrini, A.; Nobili, V. Liver stiffness in pediatric patients with fatty liver disease: Diagnostic accuracy and reproducibility of shear-wave elastography. *Radiology* **2017**, *283*, 820–827. [CrossRef] [PubMed]

13. Jung, C.; Groth, M.; Petersen, K.U.; Hammel, A.; Brinkert, F.; Grabhorn, E.; Weidemann, S.A.; Busch, J.; Adam, G.; Herrmann, J. Hepatic shear wave elastography in children under free-breathing and breath-hold conditions. *Eur. Radiol.* **2017**, *27*, 5337–5343. [CrossRef] [PubMed]

14. Ozkan, M.B.; Bilgici, M.C.; Eren, E.; Caltepe, G.; Yilmaz, G.; Kara, C.; Gun, S. Role of point shear wave elastography in the determination of the severity of fibrosis in pediatric liver diseases with pathologic correlations. *J. Ultrasound Med.* **2017**, *36*, 2337–2344. [CrossRef] [PubMed]

15. Phelps, A.; Ramachandran, R.; Courtier, J.; Perito, E.; Rosenthal, P.; MacKenzie, J.D. Ultrasound elastography: Is there a shear wave speed cutoff for pediatric liver fibrosis and inflammation? *Clin. Imaging* **2017**, *41*, 95–100. [CrossRef] [PubMed]

16. Yoon, H.M.; Kim, S.Y.; Kim, K.M.; Oh, S.H.; Ko, G.Y.; Park, Y.; Lee, J.S.; Jung, A.Y.; Cho, Y.A. Liver stiffness measured by shear-wave elastography for evaluating intrahepatic portal hypertension in children. *J. Pediatr. Gastroenterol. Nutr.* **2017**, *64*, 892–897. [CrossRef] [PubMed]

17. Behairy, B.S.; Sira, M.M.; Zalata, K.R.; Salama, E.S.E.; Abd-Allah, M.A. Transient elastography compared to liver biopsy and morphometry for predicting fibrosis in pediatric chronic liver disease: Does etiology matter? *World J. Gastroenterol.* **2016**, *22*, 4238–4249. [CrossRef] [PubMed]

18. Chen, B.; Schreiber, R.A.; Human, D.G.; Potts, J.E.; Guttman, O.R. Assessment of liver stiffness in pediatric fontan patients using transient elastography. *Can. J. Gastroenterol. Hepatol.* **2016**, *2016*. [CrossRef] [PubMed]

19. Chen, S.; Liao, B.; Zhong, Z.; Zheng, Y.; Liu, B.; Shan, Q.; Xie, X.; Zhou, L. Supersonic shearwave elastography in the assessment of liver fibrosis for postoperative patients with biliary atresia. *Sci. Rep.* **2016**, *6*, 31057. [CrossRef] [PubMed]

20. Desai, N.K.; Harney, S.; Raza, R.; Al-Ibraheemi, A.; Shillingford, N.; Mitchell, P.D.; Jonas, M.M. Comparison of controlled attenuation parameter and liver biopsy to assess hepatic steatosis in pediatric patients. *J. Pediatr.* **2016**, *173*, 160–164. [CrossRef] [PubMed]

21. Ghaffar, T.A.; Youssef, A.; Zalata, K.; ElSharkawy, A.; Mowafy, M.; Wanis, A.A.A.; Esmat, G. Noninvasive assessment of liver fibrosis in egyptian children with chronic liver diseases. *Curr. Pediatr. Res.* **2016**, *20*, 57–63.

22. Hattapoglu, S.; Goya, C.; Arslan, S.; Alan, B.; Ekici, F.; Tekbas, G.; Yildiz, I.; Hamidi, C. Evaluation of postoperative undescended testicles using point shear wave elastography in children. *Ultrasonics* **2016**, *72*, 191–194. [CrossRef] [PubMed]

23. Tokuhara, D.; Cho, Y.; Shintaku, H. Transient elastography-based liver stiffness age-dependently increases in children. *PLoS ONE* **2016**, *11*, e0166683. [CrossRef] [PubMed]

24. Belei, O.; Sporea, I.; Gradinaru-Tascau, O.; Olariu, L.; Popescu, A.; Simedrea, I.; Marginean, O. Comparison of three ultrasound based elastographic techniques in children and adolescents with chronic diffuse liver diseases. *Med. Ultrason.* **2016**, *18*, 145–150. [CrossRef] [PubMed]

25. Franchi-Abella, S.; Corno, L.; Gonzales, E.; Antoni, G.; Fabre, M.; Ducot, B.; Pariente, D.; Gennisson, J.L.; Tanter, M.; Correas, J.M. Feasibility and diagnostic accuracy of supersonic shear-wave elastography for the assessment of liver stiffness and liver fibrosis in children: A pilot study of 96 patients. *Radiology* **2016**, *278*, 554–562. [CrossRef] [PubMed]

26. Gersak, M.M.; Sorantin, E.; Windhaber, J.; Dudea, S.M.; Riccabona, M. The influence of acute physical effort on liver stiffness estimation using virtual touch quantification (VTQ). Preliminary results. *Med. Ultrason.* **2016**, *18*, 151–156. [CrossRef] [PubMed]

27. Trout, A.T.; Dillman, J.R.; Xanthakos, S.; Kohli, R.; Sprague, G.; Serai, S.; Mahley, A.D.; Podberesky, D.J. Prospective assessment of correlation between US acoustic radiation force impulse and MR elastography in a pediatric population: Dispersion of US shear-wave speed measurement matters. *Radiology* **2016**, *281*, 544–552. [CrossRef] [PubMed]

28. Mann, J.P.; De Vito, R.; Mosca, A.; Alisi, A.; Armstrong, M.J.; Raponi, M.; Baumann, U.; Nobili, V. Portal inflammation is independently associated with fibrosis and metabolic syndrome in pediatric nonalcoholic fatty liver disease. *Hepatology* **2016**, *63*, 745–753. [CrossRef] [PubMed]

29. Hanquinet, S.; Courvoisier, D.S.; Rougemont, A.L.; Wildhaber, B.E.; Merlini, L.; McLin, V.A.; Anooshiravani, M. Acoustic radiation force impulse sonography in assessing children with biliary atresia for liver transplantation. *Pediatr. Radiol.* **2016**, *46*, 1011–1016. [CrossRef] [PubMed]

30. Canas, T.; Macia, A.; Munoz-Codoceo, R.A.; Fontanilla, T.; Gonzalez-Rios, P.; Miralles, M.; Gomez-Mardones, G. Hepatic and splenic acoustic radiation force impulse shear wave velocity elastography in children with liver disease associated with cystic fibrosis. *BioMed Res. Int.* **2015**, *2015*. [CrossRef] [PubMed]

31. Dietrich, C.F.; Chichakli, M.; Hirche, T.O.; Bargon, J.; Leitzmann, P.; Wagner, T.O.; Lembcke, B. Sonographic findings of the hepatobiliary-pancreatic system in adult patients with cystic fibrosis. *J. Ultrasound Med.* **2002**, *21*, 409–416. [CrossRef] [PubMed]

32. Hanquinet, S.; Courvoisier, D.S.; Rougemont, A.L.; Dhouib, A.; Rubbia-Brandt, L.; Wildhaber, B.E.; Merlini, L.; McLin, V.A.; Anooshiravani, M. Contribution of acoustic radiation force impulse (ARFI) elastography to the ultrasound diagnosis of biliary atresia. *Pediatr. Radiol.* **2015**, *45*, 1489–1495. [CrossRef] [PubMed]

33. Dietrich, C.F.; Lorentzen, T.; Sidhu, P.S.; Jenssen, C.; Gilja, O.H.; Piscaglia, F. An introduction to the EFSUMB guidelines on interventional ultrasound (INVUS). *Ultraschall Med.* **2015**, *36*, 460–463. [CrossRef] [PubMed]

34. Lorentzen, T.; Nolsoe, C.P.; Ewertsen, C.; Nielsen, M.B.; Leen, E.; Havre, R.F.; Gritzmann, N.; Brkljacic, B.; Nurnberg, D.; Kabaalioglu, A.; et al. EFSUMB guidelines on interventional ultrasound (INVUS), part I. General aspects (long version). *Ultraschall Med.* **2015**, *36*, E1–E14. [PubMed]

35. Lorentzen, T.; Nolsoe, C.P.; Ewertsen, C.; Nielsen, M.B.; Leen, E.; Havre, R.F.; Gritzmann, N.; Brkljacic, B.; Nurnberg, D.; Kabaalioglu, A.; et al. EFSUMB guidelines on interventional ultrasound (INVUS), part I. General aspects (short version). *Ultraschall Med.* **2015**, *36*, 464–472. [PubMed]

36. Sidhu, P.S.; Brabrand, K.; Cantisani, V.; Correas, J.M.; Cui, X.W.; D'Onofrio, M.; Essig, M.; Freeman, S.; Gilja, O.H.; Gritzmann, N.; et al. EFSUMB guidelines on interventional ultrasound (INVUS), part II. Diagnostic ultrasound-guided interventional procedures (long version). *Ultraschall Med.* **2015**, *36*, E15–E35. [PubMed]

37. Sidhu, P.S.; Brabrand, K.; Cantisani, V.; Correas, J.M.; Cui, X.W.; D'Onofrio, M.; Essig, M.; Freeman, S.; Gilja, O.H.; Gritzmann, N.; et al. EFSUMB guidelines on interventional ultrasound (INVUS), part II. Diagnostic ultrasound-guided interventional procedures (short version). *Ultraschall Med.* **2015**, *36*, 566–580. [PubMed]

38. Dietrich, C.F.; Lorentzen, T.; Appelbaum, L.; Buscarini, E.; Cantisani, V.; Correas, J.M.; Cui, X.W.; D'Onofrio, M.; Gilja, O.H.; Hocke, M.; et al. EFSUMB guidelines on interventional ultrasound (INVUS), part III—abdominal treatment procedures (short version). *Ultraschall Med.* **2016**, *37*, 27–45. [CrossRef] [PubMed]

39. Dietrich, C.F.; Lorentzen, T.; Appelbaum, L.; Buscarini, E.; Cantisani, V.; Correas, J.M.; Cui, X.W.; D'Onofrio, M.; Gilja, O.H.; Hocke, M.; et al. EFSUMB guidelines on interventional ultrasound (INVUS), part III—abdominal treatment procedures (long version). *Ultraschall Med.* **2016**, *37*, E1–E32. [CrossRef] [PubMed]

40. Dietrich, C.F.; Nuernberg, D. *Interventional Ultrasound*; Thieme: Stuttgart, Germany, 2014.

41. Dietrich, C.F.; Nuernberg, D. *Interventioneller Ultraschall. Lehrbuch und Atlas für die Interventionelle Sonographie*; Thieme Verlag: Stuttgart, Germany, 2011.

42. Nobili, V.; Vizzutti, F.; Arena, U.; Abraldes, J.G.; Marra, F.; Pietrobattista, A.; Fruhwirth, R.; Marcellini, M.; Pinzani, M. Accuracy and reproducibility of transient elastography for the diagnosis of fibrosis in pediatric nonalcoholic steatohepatitis. *Hepatology* **2008**, *48*, 442–448. [CrossRef] [PubMed]

43. Kutty, S.S.; Zhang, M.; Danford, D.A.; Hasan, R.; Duncan, K.F.; Kugler, J.D.; Quiros-Tejeira, R.E.; Kutty, S. Hepatic stiffness in the bidirectional cavopulmonary circulation: The liver adult-pediatric-congenital-heart-disease dysfunction study group. *J. Thorac. Cardiovasc. Surg.* **2016**, *151*, 678–684. [CrossRef] [PubMed]

44. Berzigotti, A.; Ferraioli, G.; Bota, S.; Gilja, O.H.; Dietrich, C.F. Novel ultrasound-based methods to assess liver disease: The game has just begun. *Dig. Liver Dis.* **2018**, *50*, 107–112. [CrossRef] [PubMed]

45. Sandrin, L.; Fourquet, B.; Hasquenoph, J.M.; Yon, S.; Fournier, C.; Mal, F.; Christidis, C.; Ziol, M.; Poulet, B.; Kazemi, F.; et al. Transient elastography: A new noninvasive method for assessment of hepatic fibrosis. *Ultrasound Med. Biol.* **2003**, *29*, 1705–1713. [CrossRef] [PubMed]

46. Sigrist, R.M.S.; Liau, J.; Kaffas, A.E.; Chammas, M.C.; Willmann, J.K. Ultrasound elastography: Review of techniques and clinical applications. *Theranostics* **2017**, *7*, 1303–1329. [CrossRef] [PubMed]

47. Tsochatzis, E.A.; Gurusamy, K.S.; Ntaoula, S.; Cholongitas, E.; Davidson, B.R.; Burroughs, A.K. Elastography for the diagnosis of severity of fibrosis in chronic liver disease: A meta-analysis of diagnostic accuracy. *J. Hepatol.* **2011**, *54*, 650–659. [CrossRef] [PubMed]

48. Engelmann, G.; Gebhardt, C.; Wenning, D.; Wuhl, E.; Hoffmann, G.F.; Selmi, B.; Grulich-Henn, J.; Schenk, J.P.; Teufel, U. Feasibility study and control values of transient elastography in healthy children. *Eur. J. Pediatr.* **2012**, *171*, 353–360. [CrossRef] [PubMed]

49. De Ledinghen, V.; Le Bail, B.; Rebouissoux, L.; Fournier, C.; Foucher, J.; Miette, V.; Castera, L.; Sandrin, L.; Merrouche, W.; Lavrand, F.; et al. Liver stiffness measurement in children using fibroscan: Feasibility study and comparison with fibrotest, aspartate transaminase to platelets ratio index, and liver biopsy. *J. Pediatr. Gastroenterol. Nutr.* **2007**, *45*, 443–450. [CrossRef] [PubMed]

50. Goldschmidt, I.; Streckenbach, C.; Dingemann, C.; Pfister, E.D.; di Nanni, A.; Zapf, A.; Baumann, U. Application and limitations of transient liver elastography in children. *J. Pediatr. Gastroenterol. Nutr.* **2013**, *57*, 109–113. [CrossRef] [PubMed]

51. Lewindon, P.J.; Balouch, F.; Pereira, T.N.; Puertolas-Lopez, M.V.; Noble, C.; Wixey, J.A.; Ramm, G.A. Transient liver elastography in unsedated control children: Impact of age and intercurrent illness. *J. Paediatr. Child Health* **2016**, *52*, 637–642. [CrossRef] [PubMed]

52. Kim, S.; Kang, Y.; Lee, M.J.; Kim, M.J.; Han, S.J.; Koh, H. Points to be considered when applying fibroscan s probe in children with biliary atresia. *J. Pediatr. Gastroenterol. Nutr.* **2014**, *59*, 624–628. [CrossRef] [PubMed]

53. Alkhouri, N.; Sedki, E.; Alisi, A.; Lopez, R.; Pinzani, M.; Feldstein, A.E.; Nobili, V. Combined paediatric nafld fibrosis index and transient elastography to predict clinically significant fibrosis in children with fatty liver disease. *Liver Int.* **2013**, *33*, 79–85. [CrossRef] [PubMed]

54. Behrens, A.; Labenz, J.; Schuler, A.; Schroder, W.; Runzi, M.; Steinmann, R.U.; de Mas, C.R.; Kreuzmayr, A.; Barth, K.; Bahr, M.J.; et al. [how safe is sedation in gastrointestinal endoscopy? A multicentre analysis of 388,404 endoscopies and analysis of data from prospective registries of complications managed by members of the working group of leading hospital gastroenterologists (ALGK)]. *Z. Gastroenterol.* **2013**, *51*, 432–436. [PubMed]

55. Bernatik, T.; Schuler, A.; Kunze, G.; Mauch, M.; Dietrich, C.F.; Dirks, K.; Pachmann, C.; Borner, N.; Fellermann, K.; Menzel, J.; et al. Benefit of contrast-enhanced ultrasound (CEUS) in the follow-up care of patients with colon cancer: A prospective multicenter study. *Ultraschall Med.* **2015**, *36*, 590–593. [CrossRef] [PubMed]

56. Lee, C.K.; Perez-Atayde, A.R.; Mitchell, P.D.; Raza, R.; Afdhal, N.H.; Jonas, M.M. Serum biomarkers and transient elastography as predictors of advanced liver fibrosis in a united states cohort: The Boston children's hospital experience. *J. Pediatr.* **2013**, *163*, 1058–1064. [CrossRef] [PubMed]

57. Chongsrisawat, V.; Vejapipat, P.; Siripon, N.; Poovorawan, Y. Transient elastography for predicting esophageal/gastric varices in children with biliary atresia. *BMC Gastroenterol.* **2011**, *11*, 41. [CrossRef] [PubMed]

58. Bailey, S.S.; Youssfi, M.; Patel, M.; Hu, H.H.; Shaibi, G.Q.; Towbin, R.B. Shear-wave ultrasound elastography of the liver in normal-weight and obese children. *Acta Radiol.* **2017**, *58*, 1511–1518. [CrossRef] [PubMed]

59. Eiler, J.; Kleinholdermann, U.; Albers, D.; Dahms, J.; Hermann, F.; Behrens, C.; Luedemann, M.; Klingmueller, V.; Alzen, G.F. Standard value of ultrasound elastography using acoustic radiation force impulse imaging (ARFI) in healthy liver tissue of children and adolescents. *Ultraschall Med.* **2012**, *33*, 474–479. [CrossRef] [PubMed]

60. Hanquinet, S.; Courvoisier, D.; Kanavaki, A.; Dhouib, A.; Anooshiravani, M. Acoustic radiation force impulse imaging-normal values of liver stiffness in healthy children. *Pediatr. Radiol.* **2013**, *43*, 539–544. [CrossRef] [PubMed]

61. Matos, H.; Trindade, A.; Noruegas, M.J. Acoustic radiation force impulse imaging in paediatric patients: Normal liver values. *J. Pediatr. Gastroenterol. Nutr.* **2014**, *59*, 684–688. [CrossRef] [PubMed]

62. Fontanilla, T.; Canas, T.; Macia, A.; Alfageme, M.; Gutierrez Junquera, C.; Malalana, A.; Luz Cilleruelo, M.; Roman, E.; Miralles, M. Normal values of liver shear wave velocity in healthy children assessed by acoustic radiation force impulse imaging using a convex probe and a linear probe. *Ultrasound Med. Biol.* **2014**, *40*, 470–477. [CrossRef] [PubMed]

63. Marginean, C.O.; Marginean, C. Elastographic assessment of liver fibrosis in children: A prospective single center experience. *Eur. J. Radiol.* **2012**, *81*, e870–e874. [CrossRef] [PubMed]

64. Pinto, J.; Matos, H.; Nobre, S.; Cipriano, M.A.; Marques, M.; Pereira, J.M.; Goncalves, I.; Noruegas, M.J. Comparison of acoustic radiation force impulse/serum noninvasive markers for fibrosis prediction in liver transplant. *J. Pediatr. Gastroenterol. Nutr.* **2014**, *58*, 382–386. [CrossRef] [PubMed]

65. Tomita, H.; Hoshino, K.; Fuchimoto, Y.; Ebinuma, H.; Ohkuma, K.; Tanami, Y.; Du, W.; Masugi, Y.; Shimojima, N.; Fujino, A.; et al. Acoustic radiation force impulse imaging for assessing graft fibrosis after pediatric living donor liver transplantation: A pilot study. *Liver Transplant.* **2013**, *19*, 1202–1213. [CrossRef] [PubMed]

66. Dhyani, M.; Gee, M.S.; Misdraji, J.; Israel, E.J.; Shah, U.; Samir, A.E. Feasibility study for assessing liver fibrosis in paediatric and adolescent patients using real-time shear wave elastography. *J. Med. Imaging Radiat. Oncol.* **2015**, *59*, 687–694. [CrossRef] [PubMed]

67. Roensch, M. Lebergewebecharakterisierung Mittels Acoustic Radiation Force Impulse-Elastographie und Zone Speed Index im Kindes- und Jugendalter. Ph.D. Thesis, Martin-Luther-Universität Halle-Wittenberg, Halle, Germany, 2017.

68. Weinitschke, K. Vergleichswerterstellung für die Acoustic-Radiation-Force-Impulse-Elastographie der Leber im Kindes- und Jugendalter. Ph.D. Thesis, Martin-Luther-Universität Halle-Wittenberg, Halle, Germany, 2015.

69. Dietrich, C.F.; Nuernberg, D. *Interventional Ultrasound. A Practical Guide and Atlas*; Thieme: Stuttgart, Germany, 2014.

70. Bargon, J.; Stein, J.; Dietrich, C.F.; Muller, U.; Caspary, W.F.; Wagner, T.O. [Gastrointestinal complications of adult patients with cystic fibrosis]. *Z. Gastroenterol.* **1999**, *37*, 739–749. [PubMed]

71. Kim, J.R.; Suh, C.H.; Yoon, H.M.; Lee, J.S.; Cho, Y.A.; Jung, A.Y. The diagnostic performance of shear-wave elastography for liver fibrosis in children and adolescents: A systematic review and diagnostic meta-analysis. *Eur. Radiol.* **2018**, *28*, 1175–1186. [CrossRef] [PubMed]

72. Shin, H.J.; Kim, M.J.; Kim, H.Y.; Roh, Y.H.; Lee, M.J. Optimal acquisition number for hepatic shear wave velocity measurements in children. *PLoS ONE* **2016**, *11*, e0168758. [CrossRef] [PubMed]

73. Zhou, L.Y.; Jiang, H.; Shan, Q.Y.; Chen, D.; Lin, X.N.; Liu, B.X.; Xie, X.Y. Liver stiffness measurements with supersonic shear wave elastography in the diagnosis of biliary atresia: A comparative study with grey-scale us. *Eur. Radiol.* **2017**, *27*, 3474–3484. [CrossRef] [PubMed]

74. Hong, E.K.; Choi, Y.H.; Cheon, J.E.; Kim, W.S.; Kim, I.O.; Kang, S.Y. Accurate measurements of liver stiffness using shear wave elastography in children and young adults and the role of the stability index. *Ultrasonography* **2017**. [CrossRef] [PubMed]

75. Dong, Y.; Wang, W.P.; Xu, Y.; Cao, J.; Mao, F.; Dietrich, C.F. Point shear wave speed measurement in differentiating benign and malignant focal liver lesions. *Med. Ultrason.* **2017**, *19*, 259–264. [CrossRef] [PubMed]

76. Dietrich, C.F.; Averkiou, M.; Nielsen, M.B.; Barr, R.G.; Burns, P.N.; Calliada, F.; Cantisani, V.; Choi, B.; Chammas, M.C.; Clevert, D.A.; et al. How to perform contrast-enhanced ultrasound (CEUS). *Ultrasound Int. Open* **2018**, *4*, E2–E15. [CrossRef] [PubMed]

77. Sidhu, P.S.; Cantisani, V.; Deganello, A.; Dietrich, C.F.; Duran, C.; Franke, D.; Harkanyi, Z.; Kosiak, W.; Miele, V.; Ntoulia, A.; et al. Role of contrast-enhanced ultrasound (CEUS) in paediatric practice: An EFSUMB position statement. *Ultraschall Med.* **2017**, *38*, 33–43. [CrossRef] [PubMed]

78. Dong, Y.; Wang, W.P.; Mao, F.; Fan, M.; Ignee, A.; Serra, C.; Sparchez, Z.; Sporea, I.; Braden, B.; Dietrich, C.F. Contrast enhanced ultrasound features of hepatic cystadenoma and hepatic cystadenocarcinoma. *Scand. J. Gastroenterol.* **2017**, *52*, 365–372. [CrossRef] [PubMed]

79. Dietrich, C.F.; Dong, Y.; Froehlich, E.; Hocke, M. Dynamic contrast-enhanced endoscopic ultrasound: A quantification method. *Endosc. Ultrasound* **2017**, *6*, 12–20. [CrossRef] [PubMed]

80. Dong, Y.; Wang, W.P.; Cantisani, V.; D'Onofrio, M.; Ignee, A.; Mulazzani, L.; Saftoiu, A.; Sparchez, Z.; Sporea, I.; Dietrich, C.F. Contrast-enhanced ultrasound of histologically proven hepatic epithelioid hemangioendothelioma. *World J. Gastroenterol.* **2016**, *22*, 4741–4749. [CrossRef] [PubMed]

81. Chiorean, L.; Cui, X.W.; Tannapfel, A.; Franke, D.; Stenzel, M.; Kosiak, W.; Schreiber-Dietrich, D.; Jungert, J.; Chang, J.M.; Dietrich, C.F. Benign liver tumors in pediatric patients—Review with emphasis on imaging features. *World J. Gastroenterol.* **2015**, *21*, 8541–8561. [CrossRef] [PubMed]

82. Cui, X.W.; Pirri, C.; Ignee, A.; De Molo, C.; Hirche, T.O.; Schreiber-Dietrich, D.G.; Dietrich, C.F. Measurement of shear wave velocity using acoustic radiation force impulse imaging is not hampered by previous use of ultrasound contrast agents. *Z. Gastroenterol.* **2014**, *52*, 649–653. [CrossRef] [PubMed]

83. Piscaglia, F.; Nolsoe, C.; Dietrich, C.F.; Cosgrove, D.O.; Gilja, O.H.; Bachmann, N.M.; Albrecht, T.; Barozzi, L.; Bertolotto, M.; Catalano, O.; et al. The EFSUMB guidelines and recommendations on the clinical practice of contrast enhanced ultrasound (CEUS): Update 2011 on non-hepatic applications. *Ultraschall Med.* **2012**, *33*, 33–59. [CrossRef] [PubMed]

84. Dietrich, C.F.; Dong, Y.; Jenssen, C.; Ciaravino, V.; Hocke, M.; Wang, W.P.; Burmester, E.; Moeller, K.; Atkinson, N.S.; Capelli, P.; et al. Serous pancreatic neoplasia, data and review. *World J. Gastroenterol.* **2017**, *23*, 5567–5578. [CrossRef] [PubMed]

85. Dietrich, C.F.; Sahai, A.V.; D'Onofrio, M.; Will, U.; Arcidiacono, P.G.; Petrone, M.C.; Hocke, M.; Braden, B.; Burmester, E.; Moller, K.; et al. Differential diagnosis of small solid pancreatic lesions. *Gastrointest. Endosc.* **2016**, *84*, 933–940. [CrossRef] [PubMed]

86. Cui, X.W.; Chang, J.M.; Kan, Q.C.; Chiorean, L.; Ignee, A.; Dietrich, C.F. Endoscopic ultrasound elastography: Current status and future perspectives. *World J. Gastroenterol.* **2015**, *21*, 13212–13224. [CrossRef] [PubMed]

87. Cosgrove, D.; Barr, R.; Bojunga, J.; Cantisani, V.; Chammas, M.C.; Dighe, M.; Vinayak, S.; Xu, J.M.; Dietrich, C.F. WFUMB guidelines and recommendations on the clinical use of ultrasound elastography: Part 4. Thyroid. *Ultrasound Med. Biol.* **2017**, *43*, 4–26. [CrossRef] [PubMed]

88. Dighe, M.; Barr, R.; Bojunga, J.; Cantisani, V.; Chammas, M.C.; Cosgrove, D.; Cui, X.W.; Dong, Y.; Fenner, F.; Radzina, M.; et al. Thyroid ultrasound: State of the art. Part 2—Focal thyroid lesions. *Med. Ultrason.* **2017**, *19*, 195–210. [CrossRef] [PubMed]

89. Dighe, M.; Barr, R.; Bojunga, J.; Cantisani, V.; Chammas, M.C.; Cosgrove, D.; Cui, X.W.; Dong, Y.; Fenner, F.; Radzina, M.; et al. Thyroid ultrasound: State of the art part 1—Thyroid ultrasound reporting and diffuse thyroid diseases. *Med. Ultrason.* **2017**, *19*, 79–93. [CrossRef] [PubMed]

90. Ceyhan Bilgici, M.; Saglam, D.; Delibalta, S.; Yucel, S.; Tomak, L.; Elmali, M. Shear wave velocity of the healthy thyroid gland in children with acoustic radiation force impulse elastography. *J. Med. Ultrason.* **2018**, *45*, 75–80. [CrossRef] [PubMed]

91. Ozturk, M.; Yildirim, R. The usefulness of strain wave elastography in the diagnosis and grading of hashimoto's thyroiditis in children. *Radiol. Med.* **2017**, *122*, 960–966. [CrossRef] [PubMed]

92. Saglam, D.; Ceyhan Bilgici, M.; Kara, C.; Can Yilmaz, G.; Tanrivermis Sayit, A. Does type 1 diabetes mellitus affect the shear wave velocity of the thyroid gland of children without autoimmune thyroiditis? *Ultrasound Q.* **2017**, *33*, 225–228. [CrossRef] [PubMed]

93. Dietrich, C.F.; Bojunga, J. [Ultrasound of the thyroid]. *Laryngorhinootologie* **2016**, *95*, 87–104. [PubMed]

94. Friedrich-Rust, M.; Vorlaender, C.; Dietrich, C.F.; Kratzer, W.; Blank, W.; Schuler, A.; Broja, N.; Cui, X.W.; Herrmann, E.; Bojunga, J. Evaluation of strain elastography for differentiation of thyroid nodules: Results of a prospective degum multicenter study. *Ultraschall Med.* **2016**, *37*, 262–270. [CrossRef] [PubMed]

95. Barr, R.G.; Cosgrove, D.; Brock, M.; Cantisani, V.; Correas, J.M.; Postema, A.W.; Salomon, G.; Tsutsumi, M.; Xu, H.X.; Dietrich, C.F. WFUMB guidelines and recommendations on the clinical use of ultrasound elastography: Part 5. Prostate. *Ultrasound Med. Biol.* **2017**, *43*, 27–48. [CrossRef] [PubMed]

96. Barr, R.G.; Nakashima, K.; Amy, D.; Cosgrove, D.; Farrokh, A.; Schafer, F.; Bamber, J.C.; Castera, L.; Choi, B.I.; Chou, Y.H.; et al. WFUMB guidelines and recommendations for clinical use of ultrasound elastography: Part 2: Breast. *Ultrasound Med. Biol.* **2015**, *41*, 1148–1160. [CrossRef] [PubMed]

97. Friedrich-Rust, M.; Schwarz, A.; Ong, M.; Dries, V.; Schirmacher, P.; Herrmann, E.; Samaras, P.; Bojunga, J.; Bohle, R.M.; Zeuzem, S.; et al. Real-time tissue elastography versus fibroscan for noninvasive assessment of liver fibrosis in chronic liver disease. *Ultraschall Med.* **2009**, *30*, 478–484. [CrossRef] [PubMed]

98. Schenk, J.P.; Alzen, G.; Klingmuller, V.; Teufel, U.; El Sakka, S.; Engelmann, G.; Selmi, B. Measurement of real-time tissue elastography in a phantom model and comparison with transient elastography in pediatric patients with liver diseases. *Diagn. Interv. Radiol.* **2014**, *20*, 90–99. [PubMed]

99. Schenk, J.P.; Selmi, B.; Flechtenmacher, C.; Sakka, S.E.; Teufel, U.; Engelmann, G. Real-time tissue elastography (RTE) for noninvasive evaluation of fibrosis in liver diseases in children in comparison to liver biopsy. *J. Med. Ultrason.* **2014**, *41*, 455–462. [CrossRef] [PubMed]

100. Selmi, B.; Engelmann, G.; Teufel, U.; El Sakka, S.; Dadrich, M.; Schenk, J.P. Normal values of liver elasticity measured by real-time tissue elastography (RTE) in healthy infants and children. *J. Med. Ultrason.* **2014**, *41*, 31–38. [CrossRef] [PubMed]

101. Hermeziu, B.; Messous, D.; Fabre, M.; Munteanu, M.; Baussan, C.; Bernard, O.; Poynard, T.; Jacquemin, E. Evaluation of fibrotest-actitest in children with chronic hepatitis c virus infection. *Gastroenterol. Clin. Biol.* **2010**, *34*, 16–22. [CrossRef] [PubMed]

102. El-Shabrawi, M.H.; Mohsen, N.A.; Sherif, M.M.; El-Karaksy, H.M.; Abou-Yosef, H.; El-Sayed, H.M.; Riad, H.; Bahaa, N.; Isa, M.; El-Hennawy, A. Noninvasive assessment of hepatic fibrosis and necroinflammatory activity in egyptian children with chronic hepatitis c virus infection using fibrotest and actitest. *Eur. J. Gastroenterol. Hepatol.* **2010**, *22*, 946–951. [CrossRef] [PubMed]

103. Dietrich, C.F.; Dong, Y. Shear wave elastography with a new reliability indicator. *J. Ultrason.* **2016**, *16*, 281–287. [CrossRef] [PubMed]

104. Angulo, P.; Kleiner, D.E.; Dam-Larsen, S.; Adams, L.A.; Bjornsson, E.S.; Charatcharoenwitthaya, P.; Mills, P.R.; Keach, J.C.; Lafferty, H.D.; Stahler, A.; et al. Liver fibrosis, but no other histologic features, is associated with long-term outcomes of patients with nonalcoholic fatty liver disease. *Gastroenterology* **2015**, *149*, 389–397. [CrossRef] [PubMed]

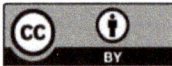

© 2018 by the authors. Licensee MDPI, Basel, Switzerland. This article is an open access article distributed under the terms and conditions of the Creative Commons Attribution (CC BY) license (http://creativecommons.org/licenses/by/4.0/).

applied sciences

MDPI

Article

A Novel Method for Assessing Regional Tendon Stiffness and Its Significance

Siu Ngor Fu [1],*, Hsing-Kuo Wang [2] and Chen Huang [1]

[1]   Department of Rehabilitation Sciences, The Hong Kong Polytechnic University, Hong Kong, China;
      amy.fu@polyu.edu.hk or cece.huang@connect.polyu.hk
[2]   School and Graduate Institute of Physical Therapy, College of Medicine, National Taiwan University,
      Center of Physical Therapy, National Taiwan University Hospital, Taipei City, Taiwan; hkwang@ntu.edu.tw
*   Correspondence: amy.fu@polyu.edu.hk; Tel.: +852-9665-1445

Received: 26 May 2018; Accepted: 27 June 2018; Published: 17 July 2018

Abstract: Elastography can be used to estimate the regional shear modulus of a tendon. This can advance our knowledge on the impact of patellar alignment and regional patellar tendon stiffness. This is important as patellar tendon abnormality is mainly found in the medial portion of the tendon in subjects with proximal patellar tendinopathy. This paper aims to assess the effect of patellar displacement on differential modulation on the shear modulus of the patellar tendon. Shear modulus is captured on the medial and lateral half of the patella tendon using the Axiplorer® ultrasound unit in conjunction with a 4–15 MHz, 50 mm linear transducer with the patellar being positioned in its resting, medio- and laterally displaced positions on 40 adults (19 females, 21 males). When the patellar is displaced laterally, the shear modulus is significantly increased at the medial half in both genders but decreased at the lateral half only in females. Conclusions: Elastography detects changes in regional tendon stiffness associated with alteration in patellar positions. The modulation on the shear modulus is gender and region specific.

Keywords: supersonic shear imaging; shear modulus; tendon stiffness; patellar positions; patellar tendon

---

1. Introduction

Supersonic shear imaging technology (SSI) is a relatively new technique to measure stiffness of soft tissue in real time [1,2]. It measures the shear wave velocity to estimate the shear modulus (an index of stiffness) of a selected area [3]. A recent study demonstrated that the tendon shear modulus generated from the SSI is correlated with the Young's modulus, which was computed from a material testing system. The study had good intra- and inter-rater reliability [4]. This new technique thereby enabled a non-invasive, direct and reliable measurement of tendon stiffness to be performed on a selected region of a tendon, providing a quantitative value. Assessment of regional tendon stiffness enabled a better understanding of mechanical demand/stress on selected regions of a tendon. This was particularly important in the patellar tendon. First, proximal patellar tendinopathy, a common knee problem, was found to have localized pathological changes, and the pathological changes were mainly detected in the medial portion of the tendon [5,6], therefore site-specific evaluation at the different regions of a tendon might have shed light on the regional changes in tissue elasticity.

The patellar tendon runs obliquely, outwardly and distally from the apex of the patella and inserts into the tibial tuberosity [7]. Patellar tendon strain could be affected by tension in the lateral retinaculum [8] or by the position of the patella [9]. Supporting this theory, a higher patellar tendon shear modulus has been associated with a higher vastus lateralis muscle shear modulus [10]. The vastus lateralis is one of the muscle heads of quadriceps femoris, which is attached to the base and the superolateral border of the patella and is connected to the lateral side of the patellar tendon through the lateral retinaculum [11]. Using magnetic resonance imaging, a trend of increased patellar lateral tilt was observed in subjects with patellar tendinopathy when compared with controls [12]. In a recent study, patellar height, as measured by the Install-Salvati ratio, was significantly greater in patients with proximal patellar tendinopathy than in healthy controls [9]. Taken together, patella mal-alignment was observed in subjects with patellar tendinopathy. The mal-alignment of the patella may have contributed to changes in the distribution of strain within the patellar tendon. Such a relationship remains to be explored. Note that increases in proximal patellar tendon stiffness have been reported in athletes with patellar tendinopathy [10,13]. The present study aimed to determine whether experimental displacement of the patella would alter patellar tendon stiffness. Regional changes in tendon stiffness were estimated using ultrasound shear wave elastography. In consideration of gender effects on patellar tendon orientation [14], both female and male subjects were recruited. We hypothesized that sideway displacement of the patella from its resting position would modulate patellar tendon shear modulus, the modulation would be site specific and greater increases in the medial half would be observed with lateral patellar displacement and in the lateral half with medial patellar displacement.

2. Materials and Methods

2.1. Ethics Statement

This study was approved by the Human Subject Ethics Subcommittee of the administrating institution. The procedures of study were fully introduced to the participants, and all of them provided their informed written consent before testing.

2.2. Participants

Forty young adults were recruited from a local university and from the community. All participants were healthy individuals aged between 18 to 30 years old and adopted a sedentary lifestyle with less than 4 h of exercise per week. Participants meeting the following criteria were excluded: (1) a past history of patellofemoral pain syndrome (PFPS); (2) previous surgeries on lower extremities; (3) any injuries altering knee alignment; (4) taking muscle-relaxation drug; (5) body mass index ≥ 30 kg/m^2.

Demographic data on age, weight, height, exercise time per week and leg dominance was recorded. The leg dominance was defined as the leg which was used to kick a ball. Quadriceps angle (q-angle) was measured as the angle formed between a line from the anterior superior iliac spine to the midpoint of patella and a vertical line joining the midpoint of patella to the tibial tubercle [15]. Because of its potential influence on the patellar tendon tension (Figure 1), the q-angle was added as a covariate factor if it was associated with changes in tendon shear modulus.

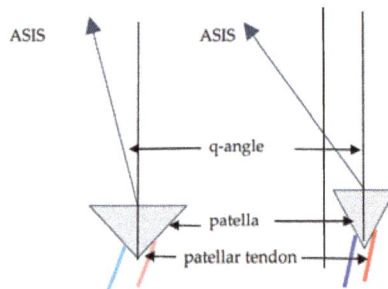

Figure 1. Relationship between the q-angle, patella and the patellar tendon. Anterior superior iliac spine and q-angle denote anterior superior iliac spine and quadriceps angle, respectively.

2.3. Procedure

Figure 2 shows the schematic flow of the study. Elastography measurement was before and after the patella was displaced from its resting position.

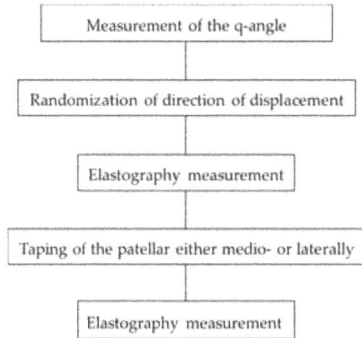

Figure 2. Schematic flow of the study.

2.3.1. Elastography Measurement

An Aixplorer® ultrasound unit (V4, Supersonic Imaging, Aix-en-Provence, France) in conjunction with a 50 mm linear-array transducer at 4–15 MHz and a frame rate up to 20,000 frames/s were used for assessing shear modulus of the patellar tendon.

Each participant was examined in supine, lying with the testing knees supported at 45° of flexion [16]. Prior to testing, subjects rested for 15 min [17]. The room temperature was controlled at 25 °C.

B-mode was used to locate and align the patellar tendon with the transducer placed longitudinal to the patellar tendon. The shear wave mode was then activated once a clear image was found. The musculoskeletal acquisition mode was used to measure the shear modulus of the patella tendon with the temporal averaging (persistence) and spatial smoothing set to medium and 6, respectively. The color-coded image was displayed, which indicated softer tissue in blue and stiffer in red. The range of color scale was pre-set from 0 to 600 kPa. The transducer was stationed on the skin with very light pressure on top of a generous amount of ultrasound gel for 8–12 s [10]. A total of five continuous ultrasound images were captured for off-line analysis with the patella of each knee being positioned in 2 positions; resting and displaced positions. The displaced direction (either medio- or laterally displaced) for the right knee was determined by drawing a card from an envelope. Once the position of the right knee had been determined, the left knee was taped in the opposite direction.

2.3.2. Patellar Positions

The patella was manually displaced towards the medial or lateral side from its resting position. Rigid tape (Strappal®, 4 cm × 10 cm) was used to hold the patella in place. The taped patella was covered by a towel so the position of the patella was blinded during SSI.

2.3.3. Data Extraction

Off-line analysis was conducted. The region of interest (ROI) was defined as a square box, which was 40 mm × 40 mm, distal to the apex of the patella. A circular quantification box (Q-Box) was centered at 0.5 cm from the apex of the patellar; and its width by the medial or lateral edge of patellar tendon from a bisecting line (Figure 3). The bisecting line was drawn from the mid-point of the cross-sectional images captured at the proximal and distal end of the patellar tendon. The medial and lateral half of the patellar tendon was defined as the patellar tendon located medio- or laterally to the bisecting line. Mean values (kPa) from the five captured imaged were computed for further analysis.

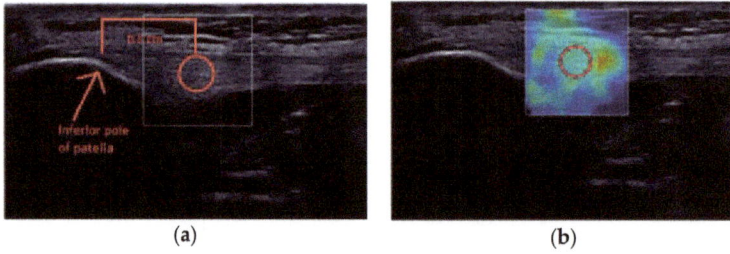

(a)   **(b)**

Figure 3. Representative images of a patellar tendon. (**a**) B-mode of the proximal patellar tendon. A 40 mm × 40 mm square box delineated the region of interest (ROI) from the apex of the patella; (**b**) shear modulus mode of the same tendon. The musculoskeletal acquisition mode was used to measure the shear modulus of the patella tendon with the temporal averaging (persistence) and spatial smoothing set to medium and 6, respectively. The color-coded image is displayed, which indicates softer tissue in blue and stiffer in red. A circular circle (Q-box) was centered at 0.5 cm from the apex of patella. Mean shear elastic modulus (kPa) of circular Q-box was computed from the system.

2.3.4. Reliability Test

The procedure was repeated on four adults (eight legs) for test-retest reliability on the same day with 30 min in-between sessions.

2.3.5. Statistical Analysis

Independent *t*-tests were performed to compare the demographic data between males and females. Intraclass correlation coefficient (ICC) was performed to analyze the test-retest reliability. Percentage changes on the tendon shear modulus were computed. Correlation coefficient tests were used in assessing the relationship between percentage change in tendon shear modulus and the q-angle measured in males and females. Repeated measures ANOVA was conducted with position (resting, displaced) and side (medial, lateral half of the patellar tendon shear modulus) as within subject factors and q-angles as co-variates if significant correlations with q-angles were detected. Statistical significance was set as $p < 0.05$. All statistical analyses were performed by SPSS version 23.0 (SPSS Inc., Chicago, IL, USA).

3. Results

3.1. Demographic Data

The age, height, weight, BMI and q-angle of participants are shown in Table 1. There were no significant differences in age and BMI between males and females ($p > 0.05$) but a significant difference was found in height, weight and q-angle between the two groups ($p = 0.001$).

Table 1. Characteristics of the participants.

Demographic	Males ($n = 21$)	Females ($n = 19$)	p
Age (year)	21.0 ± 1.9	21.8 ± 2.6	0.12
Height (cm)	173.4 ± 6.3	161.0 ± 5.1	0.001 *
Weight (kg)	63.4 ± 7.5	52.3 ± 8.1	0.001 *
Body mass index (kg/m^2)	21.1 ± 2.1	20.1 ± 2.3	0.056
q-angle (degrees)	16.9 ± 3.4	20.4 ± 3.2	0.001 *

Note: * $p < 0.05$. Data are presented as mean ± standard deviation.

3.2. Reliability Test

Test-retest reliability of patellar tendon shear modulus indicated good reliability for the lateral half (ICC = 0.94; 95% CI = 0.75 − 0.99) and medial half (ICC = 0.81; 95% CI = 0.17 − 0.96).

3.3. Effects of q-Angle on Percentage Changes in Tendon Shear Modulus

Table 2 shows that when the patella was laterally displaced, the q-angle and the percentage changes on tendon shear modulus had were positively correlated on the lateral half (r = 0.47, $p < 0.05$) but a negative correlation with the medial half (r = −0.48, $p < 0.05$) in the female subjects. No significant association was detected when the patella was displaced towards the medial side. No significant association were observed between the two variables when the patella was displaced in in the male subjects (all $p > 0.05$).

Table 2. Correlation coefficient between the q-angle and the changes in tendon shear modulus when the patella was laterally and medially displaced from its resting position.

Patella Position	Males		Females	
	Lateral Half	Medial Half	Lateral Half	Medial Half
Laterally displaced	0.29	0.17	0.47 *	−0.48 *
Medially displaced	0.01	−0.23	0.24	−0.15

Note: * $p < 0.05$.

3.4. Effect of Laterally Displaced Patellar Position on the Shear Elastic Modulus of Patellar Tendon

Table 3 lists the shear modulus when the patella was in its resting position and taped in the laterally displaced position. In the female subjects, the tendon shear modulus significantly decreased by 4% ± 39% ($p = 0.03$) in the lateral but significantly increased by 13% ± 37% ($p = 0.001$) in medial half. In male subjects, a significant increase of 17% ± 32% ($p = 0.036$) was found in the medial half of the patellar tendon. No significant change was detected in the lateral half ($p = 0.177$).

Table 3. Shear modulus of patellar tendon at its resting and displaced positions.

Patella Position	Shear modulus (KPa) Males (*n* = 20)		Shear modulus (KPa) Females (*n* = 20)	
	Lateral Half	Medial Half	Lateral Half	Medial Half
Neutral	242.1 ± 92.6	293.4 ± 85.4	281.5 ± 131.0	303.3 ± 121.8
Laterally displaced	307.9 ± 150.9	356.6 ± 147.4 *	244.3 ± 110.3 *	341.9 ± 155.1 *
Neutral	275.8 ± 104.7	341.2 ± 104.9	271.0 ± 96.8	290.7 ± 118.3
Medially displaced	280.8 ± 130.5	367.8 ± 83.4	263.3 ± 105.0	341.4 ± 140.7 *

Note: Analyses were made on patellar tendon shear modulus with the patella at its neutral and displaced positions
* $p < 0.05$.

3.5. Effect of Medially Displaced Patellar Position on the Shear Elastic Modulus of Patellar Tendon

When the patellar was taped in medially displaced position, a significant increase in the tendon shear modulus was observed in the medial half (+24 ± 35%; $p = 0.014$) with no significant change in the lateral half ($p > 0.05$) in females. No significant changes in the males were detected (Table 3, left column).

4. Discussion

Using ultrasound shear wave elastography, the present study aimed to determine the effect of patella position on regional tendon stiffness when the patella was experimentally displaced and taped from its resting position.

This was the first study exploring how patella position affects the patellar tendon shear modulus (an index of stiffness). The relationship was gender and region specific. The q-angle quantified the angle between the line of force of the quadriceps muscle and the patellar tendon. As reported in previous studies [15], we observed a greater q-angle in females than males. In addition, in the female subjects, the q-angle was positively correlated with the percentage of change in the tendon shear modulus when the patella was displaced and taped laterally. More specifically, a larger q angle was associated with a greater reduction in the tendon shear modulus on the lateral half; and a smaller increase in the shear modulus on the medial half of the patellar tendon. The male subjects exhibited a smaller q-angle, which was not correlated with the changes in tendon shear modulus when the patella was displaced. Hence, gender effects on the patellar tendon orientation may have led to tendon regional-specific adaptation and mechanical responses to patellar movement in the medio-lateral directions.

When the patella was laterally displaced, the patellar tendon became less oblique, which might have led to a reduction in tendon shear modulus. In the female subjects, a small but significant (4%) reduction in tendon shear modulus in the lateral half of the patellar tendon was detected when the patella was displaced laterally. Changes in patellar tendon obliquity would have been greater in subjects with greater q-angles. In the above paragraph, we reported the positive association between the q-angle and changes in tendon shear modulus in the lateral half of the patellar tendon. However, an increase in tendon shear modulus in the medial half in females (by 13%) and males (by 17%) was observed. The medial reticulum plays an important role as a medial stabilizer of the patella, especially at low angles and attaches onto the medial border of the patellar tendon. [18]. Increases in tension of the medial retinaculum during lateral displacement of the patella might have increased strain on the medial half of the patellar tendon. Toumi et al., 2006, noticed that the vastus medialis oblique (VMO) muscle had fibers attaching to the medial half of the patellar tendon [19]. In the present study, when the patella was taped in a laterally displaced position, increases in tension of the medial retinaculum or/and the vastus medialis oblique muscle might have led to an increase in tendon shear modulus of the medial half of the patellar tendon. Noting that the fibers of the VMO are running horizontally to the patellar tendon, its effect would be greater with the patellar tendon running vertically. Hence, subjects with smaller q-angles might have greater increases in tendon shear modulus than those with larger q-angles. The differential increase in tension at the medial and lateral half of the tendon might have induced a sheer force at the interface between the medial and lateral part of the tendon. This might have had consequences for tendon health. When the patella was displaced medially, the patellar tendon became more oblique. An increase in tendon shear modulus was expected. The changes reached a statistically significant level in the medial half in female but not male subjects. The non-significant change in male subjects might have been associated with their smaller q-angles compared with female subjects. The non-significant changes in the lateral portion were unexpected. Other factors aside from the position of the patella might have had greater effects on the lateral portion of the patellar tendon stiffness when the patella was medially displaced.

Different types of equipment, from the clinically viable to more complex systems, have been developed to estimate tendon elastic properties. The material testing system is the most direct and valid method for assessing in-vitro tendon elastic properties [20,21]. However, this method cannot be applied in-vivo. Hansen et al., 2006, proposed the use of B-mode ultrasound with a dynamometer to measure the elastic properties of human patellar tendon [22]. With this approach, ultrasound imaging was used to track tendon elongation during muscle contraction, while the muscle force was estimated from the dynamometer. This method required a long acquisition time [22]. In addition, the computed stiffness reflected the stiffness of the muscle-tendon-joint complex. Direct measurement of the tendon elastic properties was made possible with ultrasound shear wave elastography [23]. The tendon shear modulus, estimated from the ultrasound shear wave elastography techniques on patellar tendon, had good intra- and inter-rater reliability [4].

In this study, the patella was manually displaced and taped at its displaced position. We did not measure the amount of displacement and assumed that the patella would stay in place. Patellar tilting caused by medio-lateral manipulation was not considered in this study. Further studies could include measurement of patellar displacement and its effects on the modulation of tendon shear modulus. Given the relatively large variability of measurements on the tendon shear modulus, a larger sample might be warranted for further study.

5. Conclusions

Using supersonic shear imaging technology, we found gender and region-specific modulation on tendon shear modulus when the patella was displaced from its resting position. More specifically, an increase in tendon shear modulus was detected in the medial half in both genders when the patella was displaced laterally and in female subjects when the patella was medially displaced. Such findings might shed light on the pathological changes detected in the proximal and medial side of the tendinopathic tendon.

Author Contributions: Conceptualization and Methodology, S.N.F. and W.H.-K.; Investigation, C.H.; Resources, S.N.F.; Data Curation, C.H.; Writing-Original Draft Preparation, S.N.F.; Writing-Review & Editing, W.H.-K.

Funding: This research received no external funding. The Elastograph machine was donated from Lui Che Woo in establishing the LCW Special Centre for the Knee.

Acknowledgments: Francois Hug from Nante University provided valuable advice on the study idea, design and write-up. Thanks also go to Wai Lun Chu, Pak Chuen Chui, Ho Pak, Ho Yan and Tsang, Ngai Tsang for their assistance in data collection.

Conflicts of Interest: This research received no external funding.

References

1. Kot, B.C.W.; Zhang, Z.J.; Lee, A.W.C.; Leung, V.Y.F.; Fu, S.N. Elastic modulus of muscle and tendon with shear wave ultrasound elastography: Variations with different technical settings. *PLoS ONE* **2012**, *7*, e44348. [CrossRef] [PubMed]
2. Nordez, A.; Hug, F. Muscle shear elastic modulus measured using supersonic shear imaging is highly related to muscle activity level. *J Appl. Physiol.* **2010**, *108*, 1389–1394. [CrossRef] [PubMed]
3. Bercoff, J.; Tanter, M.; Fink, M. Supersonic shear imaging: A new technique for soft tissues elasticity mapping. *IEEE Trans. Ultrason. Ferroelectr. Freq. Control* **2004**, *51*, 396–409. [CrossRef] [PubMed]
4. Zhang, Z.J.; Fu, S.N. Shear elastic modulus on patellar tendon captured from supersonic shear imaging: Correlation with tangent traction modulus computed from material testing system and test–retest reliability. *PLoS ONE* **2013**, *8*, e68216. [CrossRef] [PubMed]
5. Cook, J.L.; Khan, K.M.; Kiss, Z.S.; Griffiths, L. Patellar tendinopathy in junior basketball players: A controlled clinical and ultrasonographic study of 268 patellar tendons in players aged 14-18 years. *Scand. J. Med. Sci. Sports* **2000**, *10*, 216–220. [CrossRef] [PubMed]
6. Fredberg, U.; Stengaard-Pedersen, K. Chronic tendinopathy tissue pathology, pain mechanisms, and etiology with a special focus on inflammation. *Scand. J. Med. Sci. Sports* **2008**, *18*, 3–15. [CrossRef] [PubMed]
7. Grob, K.; Manestar, M.; Filgueira, L.; Ackland, T.; Gilbey, H.; Kuster, M.S. New insight in the architecture of the quadriceps tendon. *J. Exp. Orthop.* **2006**, *3*, 32. [CrossRef] [PubMed]
8. Powers, C.M.; Chen, Y.J.; Farrokhi, S.; Lee, T.Q. Role of peripatellar retinaculum in transmission of forces within the extensor mechanism. *J. Bone Jt. Surg. Am.* **2006**, *88*, 2042–2048.
9. Crema, M.D.; Cortinas, L.G.; Lima, G.B.P.; Abdalla, R.J.; Ingham, S.J.M.; Skaf, A.Y. Magnetic Resonance imaging-based morphological and alignment assessment of the patellofemoral joint and its relationship to proximal patellar tendinopathy. *Skeletal. Radiol.* **2018**, *47*, 231–349. [CrossRef] [PubMed]
10. Zhang, Z.J.; Ng, G.Y.F.; Lee, W.C.; Fu, S.N. Increase in passive muscle tension of the quadriceps muscle heads in jumping athletes with patellar tendinopathy. *Scand. J. Med. Sci. Sports* **2017**, *27*, 1099–1104. [CrossRef] [PubMed]
11. Becker, I.; Baxter, G.D.; Woodley, S.J. The vastus lateralis muscle: An anatomical investigation. *Clin. Anat.* **2010**, *23*, 575–585. [CrossRef] [PubMed]

12. Culvenor, A.G.; Cook, J.L.; Warden, S.J.; Crossley, K.M. Infrapatellar fat pad size, but not patellar alignment, is associated with patellar tendinopathy. *Scand. J. Med. Sci. Sports* **2011**, *21*, e405–e411. [CrossRef] [PubMed]

13. Coombes, B.K.; Tucker, K.; Vicenzino, B.; Vuvan, V.; Mellor, R.; Heales, L.; Nordez, A.; Hug, F. Achilles and patellar tendinopathy display opposite changes in elastic properties: A shear wave elastography study. *Scand. J. Med. Sci. Sports* **2018**, *28*, 1201–1208. [CrossRef] [PubMed]

14. Varadarajan, K.M.; Gill, T.J.; Freiberg, A.A.; Rubash, H.E.; Li, G. Patellar tendon orientation and patellar tracking in male and female knees. *J. Orthop. Res.* **2010**, *28*, 322–328. [CrossRef] [PubMed]

15. Livingston, L.A. The quadriceps angle: A review of the literature. *J. Orthop. Sports Phys. Ther.* **1998**, *2*, 105–109. [CrossRef] [PubMed]

16. Hungerford, D.S.; Barry, M. Biomechanics of the patellofemoral joint. *Clin. Orthop. Relat. Res.* **1979**, *144*, 9–15. [CrossRef]

17. De Zordo, T.; Fink, C.; Feuchtner, G.M.; Smekal, V.; Reindl, M.; Klauser, A.S. Real-time sonoelastography findings in healthy Achilles tendons. *AJR Am. J. Roentgenol.* **2009**, *193*, W134–W138. [CrossRef] [PubMed]

18. Mitrogiannis, L.; Barbouti, A.; Kanavaros, P.; Paraskevas, G.; Kitsouli, A.; Mitrogiannis, G.; Kitsoulis, P. Cadaveric-biomechanical study on medial retinaculum: Its stabilizing role for the patella against lateral dislocation. *Folia Morphol.* **2018**. [CrossRef] [PubMed]

19. Toumi, H.; Higashiyama, I.; Suzuki, D.; Kumai, T.; Bydder, G.; McGonagle, D.; Emery, P.; Fairclough, J.; Benjamin, M. Regional variations in human patellar trabecular architecture and the structure of the proximal patellar tendon enthesis. *J. Anat.* **2006**, *208*, 47–57. [CrossRef] [PubMed]

20. Wren, T.A.; Lindsey, D.P.; Beaupre, G.S.; Carter, D.R. Effects of creep and cyclic loading on the mechanical properties and failure of human Achilles tendons. *Ann. Biomed. Eng.* **2003**, *31*, 710–721. [CrossRef] [PubMed]

21. Thambyah, A.; Thiagarajan, P.; Goh, J.C. Biomechanical study on the effect of twisted human patellar tendon. *Clin. Biomech.* **2000**, *15*, 756–760. [CrossRef]

22. Hansen, P.; Bojsen-Moller, J.; Aagaard, P.; Kjaer, M.; Magnusson, S.P. Mechanical properties of the human patellar tendon, in vivo. *Clin. Biomech.* **2006**, *21*, 54–58. [CrossRef] [PubMed]

23. Ophir, J.; Cespedes, I.; Ponnekanti, H.; Yazdi, Y.; Li, X. Elastography: A quantitative method for imaging the elasticity of biological tissues. *Ultrason. Imaging* **1991**, *13*, 111–134. [CrossRef] [PubMed]

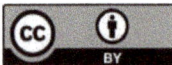

© 2018 by the authors. Licensee MDPI, Basel, Switzerland. This article is an open access article distributed under the terms and conditions of the Creative Commons Attribution (CC BY) license (http://creativecommons.org/licenses/by/4.0/).

![applied sciences logo] *applied sciences*

MDPI

Article

Shear Wave Elastography Measures of the Achilles Tendon: Influence of Time of Day, Leg Dominance and the Impact of an Acute 30-Minute Bout of Running

Catherine Payne * [iD], Peter Watt and Nick Webborn

Sport and Exercise Science and Sports Medicine Research Group, University of Brighton, Carlisle Road, Eastbourne BN20 7SN, UK; P.Watt@brighton.ac.uk (P.W.); N.Webborn@brighton.ac.uk (N.W.)
* Correspondence: c.payne2@brighton.ac.uk; Tel.: +44-1273-643754; Fax: +44-1323-745971

Received: 27 June 2018; Accepted: 16 July 2018; Published: 18 July 2018

Abstract: The mechanical properties of human tendons are likely to be influenced by factors known to affect elastic structures, including patterns of loading and unloading during the day. However, the exact scale and relevance of these variables to tendon stiffness remains unclear. The aim of this study was to (1) measure Achilles tendon (AT) stiffness over the course of the day, (2) examine AT stiffness between dominant and non-dominant standing leg tendons and (3) assess the impact of previous activity on AT stiffness. To assess the impact of time of day and leg dominance, 15 healthy participants (6 females, 9 males; mean age 28 ± 4 year, mean VISA-A score 99.0 ± 1.2) had shear wave elastography (SWE) measures taken at 08:00 h, 12:30 h and 17:00 h on both dominant and non-dominant legs. To assess the impact of exercise, 24 tendons were analysed (7 females, 5 males; mean age 27 ± 4 year, mean VISA-A Score 99.1 ± 1.1) with participants randomly assigned to either a control (CONT) group or a running (RUN) group. The RUN group performed a 30-min run at a subjective intensity of 13–15 on rating of perceived exertion (RPE) scale and had SWE measures taken before, immediately after, 6 h 24 h, 48 h and 72 h following the run. There were no significant differences in AT stiffness over the course of a day or between dominant and non-dominant leg. Significant increases in AT stiffness were noted pre-post run (0.27 m/s, 2.95%, $p = 0.037$). Leg dominance does not affect SWE values from asymptomatic ATs or change throughout a day, but a 30-min run significantly increases AT stiffness. Leg dominance and timing of clinical appointments are unlikely to affect SWE results, however a prior bout of physical activity may cause changes within the AT resulting in a significantly different SWE measure. Clinicians and researchers should be cautious of interpreting SWE results if weight bearing exercise has been performed beforehand.

Keywords: Achilles tendon; shear wave elastography; ultrasound elastography; time of day; leg dominance; prior activity

---

1. Introduction

The mechanical properties of human tendons are likely to be influenced by factors known to affect elastic structures, including patterns of loading and unloading during the day. The scale and relevance of these variables to tendon structure and function remain relatively unclear [1] and there are few systematic reports on how the stiffness of a human tendon alters throughout the course of a day [2,3]. Periods of sleep, rest and activity throughout a day will cause altered loading and unloading at differing frequencies and intensities on tendons, which will impact their stiffness. The research available into the effect of time of day on tendon structures in vivo has been conducted using the patella tendon, with tendon stiffness estimated using an isokinetic dynamometer to measure force and B-mode ultrasound to measure length [2]. This research measured a decrease in tendon stiffness of 20.2 ± 9.5% between the testing times of 08:00 h and 18:00 h [2]. No research has yet assessed the impact of time of day on tendon stiffness using shear wave elastography (SWE).

The term mechanotransduction refers to the processes converting mechanical loading, such as exercise, into measurable cellular responses that may result in structural or functional change [4]. Exercise has been shown capable of altering both the structural and chemical makeup of human tendon by inducing increases in its cross-sectional area and increasing the concentration of metabolic enzymes to increase collagen turnover and prostaglandin production [5,6]. Mechanical stimulus is also postulated to initiate changes within the extracellular matrix of tendon that results in a more damage resistant tissue with optimal force transmission properties [7]. The early adaptive responses to mechanotransduction can initiate longer term alterations in the mechanical properties of a tendon [8], however the majority of alterations brought about by mechanotransduction are noted as the result of repeated exercise (loading) programmes. This could be because the adaptation in the mechanical properties of tendons takes a long time, or the impact of acute bouts of exercise have not yet been extensively studied. Regardless, the exact influence of acute bouts of specific forms of exercise on the mechanical properties of healthy human tendon remains relatively unclear [1,9]. Long term exercise training such as running may increase the mass, collagen content, ultimate tensile strength and load to failure of a tendon [5], but changes in relation to acute exercise bouts are less well understood.

A systematic review of the immediate effect of exercise on AT properties was conducted in 2013 [10]. The conclusion of this paper was that acute bouts of exercise impact AT mechanical properties in a manner dependent on both mode and dose of exercise as the differences in tendon stress-strain characteristics, such as rate, duration and frequency, between different types of exercise will cause varying changes to the mechanical properties of tendons over time [10]. Of the papers included in the review by Obst et al. (2013), 14 assessed AT stiffness with 12 of these using data obtained from ultrasonography and dynamometry [11–22]. Whilst the remaining two studies also utilised ultrasonography, they used either a force platform or a force transducer to obtain measures of force [23,24]. Six papers reported a decrease in AT stiffness following exercise, one reported a significant increase and the remaining seven reported no differences [10]. Of the articles that found a decrease in AT stiffness, four assessed the effect of stretching, whilst others assessed isometric or concentric muscle contractions and not specifically running. One study found a significant increase in tendon stiffness post 10 minutes of static stretching with stiffness calculated using ultrasonography and isokinetic dynamometry [18]. Only two articles included in the review assessed tendon stiffness after running, one study found no difference in AT stiffness post running [23]. The other study found no significant difference in stiffness, however, it only looked at changes after a 6-min warm up jog and stretching [19]. Also noted in the Obst et al. (2013) paper was the lack of studies evaluating the mechanical properties of the 'free' AT [10], with 'free' AT referring to the part of the tendon without any other attachment to either bony or muscular structures. This current study therefore aims to focus on the 'free' portion of the AT to address this gap in the literature.

Although not directly assessing stiffness, research using ultrasound tissue characterisation (UTC) has assessed the structure of the human in vivo AT before and after exercise. The results of studies using UTC suggest there were changes in tendon structure and integrity following a bout of exercise, including a decrease in aligned tendon fibrils and an increase in the separation and waviness of fibrils, both of which returned to baseline over the following 72 h [25]. A decrease in the alignment of the tendon fibres may result in decreased tendon stiffness. Habitual running of long distances (>80 km/week for >3 years) results in a marked increase in the cross-sectional area of the AT of approximately 22% in comparison with a non-running control group [26]. This increase in cross-sectional area may be a compensatory mechanism as pathological tendons can compensate for significant areas of disorganised fibres by increasing thickness to reduce stress and maintain structural homeostasis to ensure adequate load bearing [27,28]. Despite a large body of work surrounding the effects of habitual running, studies exploring the impact of a single acute bout of running on stiffness measures of normal, healthy human ATs in vivo remain scarce [10,19].

Most research into tendon stiffness utilise direct methods of calculating stiffness using ultrasound to measure change in tendon length and a dynamometer to measure force. This can produce accurate results, but is time consuming, requires complex procedures and a lot of equipment and space to run. Hence, a quick, easy and non-invasive measure of tendon stiffness is required. This study proposes to measure shear wave velocity (SWV), a surrogate measure of stiffness, in the AT in vivo using shear wave elastography (SWE). The relatively recent introduction of SWE offers a novel way to quantitatively assess tendon stiffness by measuring SWV through a tissue, providing information on tissue stiffness [29]. In recent years, there have been several studies published using SWE to assess tendon stiffness [30–34] and many reporting the reliability and validity of SWE [33,35,36]. Despite this, the reported information on the many variables that potentially influence SWE measurements remain unclear [32]. It is necessary to understand normal variation in AT stiffness with relation to leg dominance [37], as ATs have been shown to be significantly different between dominant and non-dominant legs [38] having different mechanical properties attributed to different loading profiles of both legs during daily activity due to foot dominance [39]. No studies have examined differences in AT stiffness with leg dominance using SWE or the alterations in SWE measurements experienced within a healthy human AT in vivo, in response to the time of day or an acute bout of running.

It is important to understand the normal variation in SWV measures within the AT in vivo and the influence of external loads on these values. Without such information, abnormal or clinically relevant values cannot be decided upon and accurate interpretation is not possible. The aim of this study is three-fold. Firstly, it will measure the stiffness of the AT using SWE in the morning (08:00 h), afternoon (12:30 h) and evening (17:00 h) to see whether any measurable differences are apparent dependent on time of day. Secondly, it will examine SWE measures obtained in ATs in vivo bi-laterally to assess measurable differences between dominant and non-dominant standing leg tendons. Thirdly, this study will use SWE to assess measures of stiffness taken before, immediately after, 6 h, 24 h, 48 h and 72 h after an acute 30-min bout of running to trace the time course of SWV alterations in the AT in vivo after exercise.

2. Materials and Methods

2.1. Participants

To assess the impact of time of day and leg dominance, 15 healthy participants were examined (6 females, 9 males; mean age 28 ± 4 year, mean VISA-A score 99.0 ± 1.2). To determine foot dominance, participants were asked to identify which foot they would kick a ball with [40–42]. To assess the impact of a 30-min bout of running, 24 tendons from 12 participants were analysed (7 females, 5 males; mean age 27 ± 4 year, mean VISA-A Score 99.1 ± 1.1). Inclusion criteria was set as both males and females over the age of 18 years old who achieved a minimum score of 96/100 on the VISA-A to rule out subjectively symptomatic tendons. Exclusion criteria included previous diagnosis of Achilles tendinopathy, history of pain in the AT area lasting for more than 24 h, pregnancy, previous medical or surgical intervention on the AT or abnormal features consistent with Achilles Tendinopathy on conventional 2D ultrasound.

Participants were recruited by word of mouth from the University department where the testing took place. All participants provided written informed consent to participate in the study and all procedures performed involving human participants were commenced following ethical approval for the study being obtained from the University of Brighton ethics committee, in line with the 1964 Helsinki declaration and its later amendments.

2.2. Methods

To assess the impact of time of day, all participants were scanned three times throughout the course of their normal working day. Firstly, between 08:00–08:30 h, secondly between 12:30–13:00 h and lastly between 17:00–17:30 h. To assess the impact of leg dominance, SWE measures were taken on both the dominant and non-dominant legs. Participants were asked to maintain any daily walking activity they deemed normal but refrain from any other exercise for 48 h before testing and during the testing period.

To assess the impact of an acute bout of running, participants were randomly placed into the intervention group of running (RUN) or the control (CONT) group. If assigned to the CONT group, participants were asked to remain seated in the examination room for a period of at least 30 min, and no more than 40 min during their testing session. The participants were asked to remain seated keeping their legs still during this period and not move around, the experimenter was always present to ensure this occurred. Following assignment to each intervention group, the measures outlined below were taken from each participant immediately before and immediately after their sitting or running intervention. Subsequent follow up measures were also taken at 6 h, 24 h, 48 h and 72 h post intervention. In the RUN group, participants were given the possibility to warm up on the treadmill for no more than 5 min. Following the warm up, they were asked to keep the incline on the treadmill at 1% and increase the speed of the treadmill to a pace they felt comfortable with, and to run for a period of 30 min. A Rating of Perceived Exertion (RPE) scale [43] was placed in the direct eye line of the participants and they were asked to maintain an RPE of at least 13 (representing an intensity of somewhat hard), but below 15 (hard). The participants were asked every 5 min to rate their current RPE value and were encouraged by the experimenter to maintain an RPE of between 13 and 15 if it was outside of these values. The participants were able to alter their speed during their 30-min run to maintain RPE between these boundaries. Following 30 min of running, participants could complete a cool down at a walking speed of their choice for a period of no more than 5 min.

2.3. Scanning Techniques

During all measures, participants lay prone with both feet hanging clear of an examination table and an amount of ultrasound gel sufficient to maintain good contact between the ultrasound probe and the skin was applied. All measures were taken with a Siemens ACUSON S3000™ HELX EVOLUTION Ultrasound System (Siemens Medical Solutions, Mountain View, CA, USA). Measures obtained were shear wave velocity (SWV) which was used for analysis without converting to Young's modulus.

2.4. Conventional Ultrasound Technique

During each measurement, extended field of view 'SieScape' images were taken on grey scale ultrasound by a single operator (CP), with three years imaging experience, using a 14L5SP probe to visualize the 'free' AT length, between insertion of the AT the calcaneus to the lowest fibres of soleus, following previous methodology [44]. Tendon mid-point was calculated as half AT length and used as the reference point for all subsequent measures to ensure all were taken at the tendon mid-point, relative to each participant.

Measures of maximum anterior-posterior (max AP) diameter were calculated at the tendon mid-point relative to each participant using a 14L5 probe. A transverse image of the AT was captured from the tendon mid-point and the ultrasound software used to measure the maximum distance in millimetres (mm) from the anterior border of the tendon to the posterior border of the tendon. As used in previous research [45], three consecutive measures were taken, ensuring all measures fell within 5 mm of each other, with the mean of the three measurements taken to represent max AP diameter.

2.5. Shear Wave Elastography

Following conventional ultrasound, the system was placed into Virtual Touch IQ (VTIQ) mode, an acoustic radiation force-based method that produces both qualitative and quantitative maps of SWV ranging between 0.5 and 10.0 m/s [46,47]. Images were obtained by the same operator (CP) using a linear-array 9L4 transducer probe. Due to the saturation limit of the technology, a SWV value measured above 10 m/s was returned by the software as 'High'. Only 4 of these were returned throughout the course of the study and when they did occur, they were discounted from the study. Image quality was closely monitored throughout examination, tissue compression was avoided. Quality maps were assessed to ensure images conformed to a high level of quality, specifically checking for a quality map all green in colour, which indicates that a correct amount of pressure was used. All elastograms were taken in a longitudinal plane with the foot in a relaxed foot position, as this has been demonstrated to provide the most reproducible measures [44].

Ten set size and shape regions of interest (ROI) were placed manually in the same order on longitudinal elastograms, at a standardised depth of 0.5 cm, along the tendon length, starting proximally and working distally (See Figure 1).

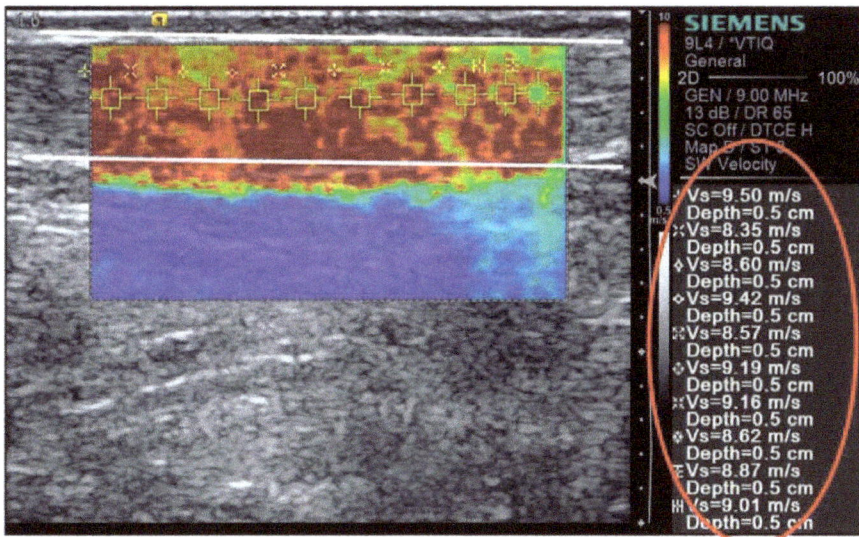

Figure 1. Longitudinal shear wave elastogram of the right Achilles tendon taken from a 24-year-old male participant. The image shows 10 regions of interest (ROI's) used to collect shear wave elastography data with the corresponding values in m/s shown to the right of the image highlighted in the red circle.

2.6. Statistical Analysis

All statistical analysis was performed using SPSS version 22 (SPSS, Chicago, IL, USA.). Basic measurements of the participants were expressed as mean ± standard deviation. Distribution of groups was analysed using the Shapiro-Wilk test. A one-way repeated measures ANOVA assessed any change to SWV over the three measured time points. A paired sample t-tests was used to examine whether measures taken on the dominant and non-dominant sides of the participants were significantly different from each other. A two-way repeated measures ANOVA (Time (6) and Group (2)) assessed differences in SWV following exercise. To establish where the differences lay, separate one-way repeated measures ANOVA's were completed for the RUN and CONT groups with findings followed up using the Bonferonni post hoc test. Data was checked for sphericity with the Huynh-Feldt correction applied if necessary and alpha level was set at $p < 0.05$ throughout.

3. Results

3.1. Time of Day

There were no significant differences shown to exist over the three measured time points for either AT length ($p = 0.411$) or max AP diameter ($p = 0.286$) in the dominant ATs or in the non-dominant ATs ($p = 0.062$ and $p = 0.322$, respectively).

In relation to time of day, there were no significant differences ($p > 0.05$) over the three measured time points in the SWV within either the participants' dominant AT ($p = 0.094$) or non-dominant AT ($p = 0.143$). Alterations in the group mean of the SWV measures within the dominant AT did not experience significant alterations throughout the day. There was a small reduction in measured stiffness throughout the morning, between 08:00 h and 12:30 h of -2.07% and an increase between 12:30 h and 17:00 h of 0.63%. Overall, between 08:00–17:00 h, the decrease in SWV was -1.45%. None of these alterations were shown to be significant.

3.2. Leg Dominance

When compared to each other, there were no significant differences between dominant and non-dominant ATs with regards to AT length at 08:00 h ($p = 0.789$), 12:30 h ($p = 0.718$) or 17:00 h ($p = 0.727$). There were no significant differences between dominant and non-dominant ATs with regards to AT max AP diameter at 08:00 h ($p = 0.608$), 12:30 h ($p = 0.681$) or 17:00 h ($p = 0.714$). There were no significant differences in the SWV measures in the dominant AT compared to the non-dominant AT ($p > 0.05$) at 08:00 h ($p = 0.176$), 12:30 h ($p = 0.402$) and 17:00 h ($p = 0.915$). The mean SWV measured in the dominant AT of both male (mean = 9.61 ± 0.21; range 9.24–9.88 m/s) and female (mean = 9.76 ± 0.23; range 9.31–9.92 m/s) participants were very similar ($p = 0.203$) indicating no significant differences between the SWE measures within the AT of male and female participants.

3.3. Acute Bout of Exercise

The basic measurements obtained from the participants over the measured time points are displayed in Table 1.

Table 1. AT Length (mm), AT maximum anterior-posterior (Max A-P) diameter (mm) and SWV at all measured time points for both RUN and CONT group.

	PRE	POST	6 h POST	24 h POST	48 h POST	72 h POST
RUN AT Length (mm)	44.3 ± 11.2	45.0 ± 11.2	44.8 ± 11.3	44.1 ± 11.1	44.3 ± 11.1	44.1 ± 10.8
CONT AT Length (mm)	29.9 ± 5.7	29.6 ± 6.2	30.0 ± 5.9	30.0 ± 5.6	30.2 ± 5.6	30.0 ± 5.2
RUN Max AP (mm)	4.37 ± 0.27	4.08 ± 0.19	4.58 ± 0.29	4.38 ± 0.26	4.45 ± 0.31	4.34 ± 0.28
CONT Max AP (mm)	4.66 ± 0.64	4.69 ± 0.63	4.63 ± 0.64	4.71 ± 0.61	4.63 ± 0.69	4.66 ± 0.63
RUN SWV (m/s)	9.16 ± 0.39	9.43 ± 0.39	9.00 ± 0.42	9.19 ± 0.31	9.04 ± 0.36	9.05 ± 0.28
CONT SWV (m/s)	9.11 ± 0.23	9.08 ± 0.22	9.04 ± 0.26	9.05 ± 0.22	9.06 ± 0.21	9.09 ± 0.22

When considering the effect of the exercise bout, measurements of AT length for both the RUN and the CONT group remain stable over the six measured time points with no significant differences apparent over time ($p > 0.05$). In the CONT group, no significant differences occurred over the time points for either max AP or SWV. In contrast, the RUN group experienced significant changes ($p < 0.05$) in max AP and SWV.

The results demonstrated significant differences in the data for the RUN group in relation to the max AP diameter. The absolute difference, % difference and the significance of the significant differences in max AP diameter are shown in Table 2.

Table 2. Absolute difference, % difference and p value for the significant differences shown in max AP diameter. * = $p < 0.05$, ** = $p < 0.01$.

	Absolute Difference	% Difference	Significance
Pre-Post	−0.29 mm	−6.64%	$p = 0.000$ **
Pre-6 h	0.21 mm	4.81%	$p = 0.042$ *
Post-6 h	0.50 mm	12.25%	$p = 0.000$ **
Post-24 h	0.30 mm	7.35%	$p = 0.000$ **
Post-48 h	0.37 mm	9.07%	$p = 0.000$ **
Post-72 h	0.26 mm	6.37%	$p = 0.000$ **
Post-6 h–Post-24 h	−0.20 mm	−4.37%	$p = 0.028$ *

With regards to measures of SWV, the results demonstrated a significant main effect of Time ($p = 0.001$), no significant differences between the groups ($p > 0.05$) but a significant interaction effect of time × group ($p = 0.003$), implying a significant difference between the measured time points depending on which group a participant was in. The absolute differences and significance values for the SWV data is shown in Table 3 and the mean alterations in SWV for the RUN group are shown in Figure 2. There were no significant differences in the time points for the CONT group ($p = 0.614$) implying that the SWV data collected for all the participants in the CONT group did not vary significantly over the measured time points and therefore remained stable.

Table 3. Absolute difference, % difference and p value for the significant differences shown in SWV. * = $p < 0.05$.

	Absolute Difference	% Difference	Significance
Pre-Post	−0.27 m/s	−2.95%	$P = 0.037$ *
Post-6 h	−0.43 m/s	−4.56%	$P = 0.019$ *
Post-48 h	−0.39 m/s	−4.14%	$P = 0.015$ *
Post-72 h	−0.38 m/s	−4.03%	$P = 0.013$ *

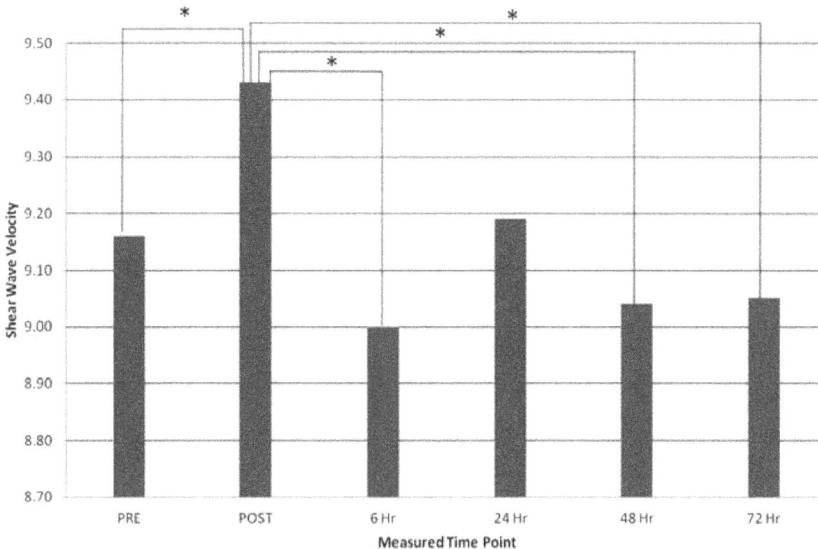

Figure 2. Alterations in average SWV measures in the RUN group over the measured time points with significant differences included. * = $p < 0.05$.

The largest changes in the SWV values were in the RUN group where SWV increased pre-post by 0.27 m/s (2.95%). After this, the SWV decreased by approximately -4.5%, before once again increasing by just over 2%. In contrast to the above changes noted in the RUN group, the largest percentage change experienced in the CONT group was just 0.44%. If considering all the measured time points in relation to the PRE-values, the largest change again was an almost 3% increase measured in the RUN group between pre and post. However, as the POST measure is the only measure to be significantly different from PRE, it would suggest that the SWV measures return to normal after a period of 6 h following an acute 30-min bout of running. The mean increase in SWV following the exercise bout was 0.27 m/s, followed by a decrease between the post measure and 6 h measure of -0.43 m/s with the range of increase being between 0.05–0.81 m/s.

The largest changes in the SWV values were in the RUN group in the POST measure which was taken immediately after the 30 min run, with SWV increasing by 0.27 m/s (2.95%). The SWV value appears to rise immediately after exercise followed by a compensatory drop of -0.43 m/s (-4.56%), 6 h after exercise compared to the measure taken at POST. The SWV measure in the RUN group taken at 6 h post exercise is below that taken prior to exercise (as seen in Figure 1), but as it is not significantly different from the PRE value, it can be said that SWV values return to baseline levels after a period of 6 h following 30-min of running.

4. Discussion

This study is the first to trace the stiffness of the human AT in vivo over the course of a normal working day using SWE and to compare SWE results between dominant and non-dominant legs. This study also examined whether an acute bout of running for a period of 30 min leads to any significant alterations in SWV values experienced in the AT in vivo as measured using SWE. The main findings of this study advance our understanding of SWE by showing that measures taken on healthy asymptomatic ATs experience no significant alterations in the SWV (and hence stiffness) measured in either the dominant or non-dominant AT of participants. The data also demonstrates that healthy ATs do not experience significant alterations in SWV (and hence stiffness) throughout the day indicating that time of day does not need to be considered when performing repeated scans of the AT in varying clinic appointment times. Our data also provides clear evidence that in comparison to a control group, a significant increase in SWV was apparent immediately after a 30 min run. The implications of these results are that a prior bout of physical activity may initiate changes within the physical properties of the AT that could result in a significantly different SWV measure. A clinician should be aware of the possibility of obtaining a significantly increased SWV measure from the AT using SWE if 30 min of weight bearing exercise has been performed within the previous 6 h. The responses to longer periods of tendon loading on SWV, and its time course have not been investigated and may merit further enquiry.

The purpose of assessing the impact of time of day on SWE measures was to examine whether time of day should be considered when performing repeated scans of the AT for diagnosis or during treatment. Although this study did not encompass a whole 24 h period, it does relate directly to times where most clinical assessment is likely to occur, providing direct significance for the clinical usage of SWE. This study examined the SWV experienced within healthy, asymptomatic ATs over the course of a working day using times similar to those used in previous research [2,3], with measures taken at 08:00 h, 12:30 h and 17:00 h. This study explicitly controlled for out of the ordinary, intense/heavy exercise both before and during the testing period and allowed insight into stiffness changes throughout the day. The results of this study will be important when considering the use of SWE for both early diagnosis and monitoring of recovery, which would likely have a clinical impact on not only long-term rehabilitation but also return to activities, specifically in high-level athletes [33].

Previous research has reported decreases in tendon stiffness throughout the course of the day to the magnitude of 20.2% and 21% [2,3]. It was hypothesised these decreases in stiffness were attributed to either hormonal changes or the action of general mobilisation throughout the day [2]. The results of this study however, were markedly different, with the individual changes showing no systematic change in stiffness and the magnitude of change in tendon stiffness was only approximately 2%. These changes were not statistically significant and therefore this study can report no change in tendon stiffness with time of day. The decrease in tendon stiffness noted above, between morning and evening, was only shown to be true when tendon stiffness was calculated at low force levels (calculated from the gradient of the tangent over force levels corresponding to 1205N). However, when tendon stiffness was calculated a high force levels (100% MVC), there was no significant change noted between morning and evening ($p = 0.10$). This finding was potentially attributed to the fact that when measured during MVC, the tendon was stretched to a position on its curve where stiffness is highest [2]. Differences between the previous research and this study which may provide some rationale for the differences in findings include the tendon being examined (patella vs AT), the method of obtaining stiffness measures (ultrasonography and isokinetic dynamometer vs SWE) and differences in populations studies (purely male cohort vs mixed sex cohort). SWE as a methodology has been validated against traditional tensile testing [36] and the results of this study showed no significant differences between the SWV of males and females, so the use of a differing cohort should not impact the results.

To assess the effect of leg dominance on SWE measures of the AT, the dominant and non-dominant ATs of each participant were identified [38], with the majority of people identifying their right foot as being dominant [39]. As an association between full rupture in the AT and micro-tear formation has been previously shown, it would indicate that the ATs of the dominant side will be more at risk of both micro-tear and full rupture [48]. This increase in micro-tears is hypothesised to result in tendon hypertrophy as the tendon constantly repairs and remodels itself [48], which would explain a higher cross-sectional area of tendon noted in athletes compared to the general population [26]. An increased thickness can also be a result of short-term injury which can result in tendon thickening in an attempt to reduce stress [28].

Some research has shown no significant variation in the length of the AT between dominant and non-dominant ankles [38], however in contrast, other authors have found the length of the free AT of the dominant leg to be significantly greater than the non-dominant leg [39]. These two studies also differ in their findings in relation to the cross-sectional area of the AT. One study found no significant difference in the average cross-sectional area of the free AT between legs [39] whereas others demonstrate cross-sectional area to be significantly larger in dominant ankles [38], which can impact stiffness. The Bohm et al. (2015) reported no significant differences between the sides in tendon stiffness (N/mm) [39] as found in this current study. In the present study, no noted significant differences ($p > 0.05$) in stiffness measures were obtained with SWE were found in healthy, asymptomatic subjects with no history of symptomatic Achilles tendinopathy, between dominant and non-dominant tendons.

The mean increase in SWV following the exercise bout was 0.27 m/s with the range of increase for all participants being between 0.05–0.81 m/s. This was followed by a decrease between the post measure and 6 h measure of −0.43 m/s. These alterations were shown to be statistically significant, therefore just 30 min of running was shown to significantly increase SWV by 0.27 m/s, and therefore increase AT stiffness. Studies using UTC have shown that exercise leads to a change in tendon structure in both race horses and humans [25,49] when tendons were measured prior to the bout of exercise, then again one, two and four days after the exercise bout. Changes in the structure of the tendon may be expected to affect its mechanical properties, e.g., tendon stiffness and this study adds some support to that notion as exercise resulted in a significantly increased measure of SWV, even after an acute bout of exercise lasting 30 min. In the UTC study involving human participants, the authors concluded that exercise resulted in a short-duration (72 h period) and fully reversible response of the tendon which occurred with no loss of integrity of the collagen matrix [25]. Alterations in the extra-cellular matrix of the tendon including an increase in cytoplasmic organelles for increased protein production, in particular proteoglycans, which are associated with an increase in bound water can result in an increase in cross-sectional area after exercise [28]. This study however, demonstrated that a 30-min acute bout of running exercise resulted in a decrease in maximum anterior-posterior tendon thickness (mm) following an acute bout of exercise. This decrease in tendon thickness has also been shown in other research and hypothesised to be attributed to a loss of fluid from the tendon to the peritendinous space caused by the mechanical load inducing increased hydrostatic pressure [10]. This temporary 'dehydration' within the tendon could be a potential cause of differences found in SWV, as it may affect tissue density.

Alterations in tendon mechanical properties including increases in stiffness may be the bodies response to a new level of loading and potentially aid in reducing tendon damage caused by mechanical fatigue [50]. An increased level of stiffness detected immediately after an acute mechanical load, may allow for less extension of the tendon [50] which potentially may help reduce macro-trauma risk. Previous research demonstrated that in young healthy ATs, an acute bout of eccentric exercise resulted in a significant increase in AT stiffness as measured with SWE [51]. Other studies however show that a single 30-min bout of running did not impact the stiffness of the AT and concluded that the mechanical properties of tendons remain constant throughout locomotion [23]. The research of Farris et al. utilised the same number of participants as in this study, but required participants to complete a 30-min run at a set pace of 12 km/ph. This speed was selected as being representative of a recreational run, as all participants said they were recreational runners, therefore the speed of the run between these studies could have varied. In contrast to Farris et al., this study utilised a self-paced run, asking participants to maintain an RPE level between 13–15 to ensure the run was the same subjective intensity for all participants. The mechanical properties of the ATs of each subject in the Farris study were recorded both before and after the run during a series of hops, with tendon stiffness estimated using the traditional format using AT length data obtained using an ultrasound probe secured to the participants leg using bandaging tape and AT force as measured using force plates [23]. In contrast, this study utilised SWE. Reductions in tendon stiffness following unaccustomed acute bouts of exercise may increase injury risk [10], however the participants in this study all self-reported as being moderately active on a regular basis in activities that involved running, and who therefore should have been accustomed to this dose and manner of exercise used.

This study is the first to use SWE to trace alterations in AT stiffness in vivo over the course of a day, the first to compare AT stiffness between dominant and non-dominant standing leg ATs and the first to use SWE to assess alterations in AT stiffness in vivo following an acute bout of running. As with all studies, it does carry some limitations including a saturation limit to the measures the Siemens ACUSON S3000™ HELX EVOLUTION Ultrasound System (Siemens Medical Solutions, USA) can obtain. SWVs above 10 m/s simply return a value of 'High'. Although there were very few 'High' values noted throughout data collection, it is not possible to say how fast the SWV was for these measures, therefore any measures returned as 'High' were discounted from the study. This study examined variation in the AT of 15 healthy subjects to assess leg dominance and time of day, based on the numbers used in previous literature (range 8–12 subjects) as a guideline [2,3,52]. The impact of these variables on SWE data has not been previously examined and therefore replicating the number of subjects from previous research was the best starting place. The impact of exercise on SWE measures has also not been previously studied and therefore it is not possible to complete an accurate power analysis. Therefore 12 participants were analysed, to match the number used in very similar research [23]. However, this leads to a limitation of the study, that is, the use of a relatively small homogenous sample. Despite this, 10 data points (ROIs) were taken from each elastogram at each testing session and there were three testing sessions in the time of day section (08:00 h, 12:00 h and 17:00 h) and six in the exercise section. Therefore, the total numbers of measures taken from all participants over the course of the testing and included in the analysis for this study is over 1500 measures, a number much higher than that used in previous research. All participants were considered healthy and free of lower limb injury. This was considered important as until the normal variations within healthy tendons are established and some baseline clinical values recorded, it will be impossible to establish what is normal, acceptable change, versus pathological change and therefore, of concern. It is however not possible to generalize the results from this study to any symptomatic individuals with pathology or who fall outside the tested age range. Future research should define other populations based on age, sex or other covariates expected to influence stiffness as well as examining the results obtained from pathological samples. It is worth noting here the limitations of SWE with regards to anisotropy, as SWE utilises ultrasound to trace the propagation of generated shear waves, so with ultrasound scanning, a controlled angle of the transducer to the skin is crucial in obtaining an accurate image and obtaining reliable values for SWE. Shear waves propagate more readily along longitudinal fibres than they do across them [36] and therefore it has been noted that the transducer for SWE should be orientated parallel to the direction of the fibres being assessed to ensure the most accurate results [53]. Our own previous work [54] also demonstrated that certain protocols can be utilised when using SWE to assess the stiffness of the human Achilles tendon in vivo to standardise the measurements and obtain the most accurate results. These include using longitudinal images and keeping the foot in a relaxed position whilst scanning.

The exercise mode utilised in this study was running, however other modes of exercise such as stretching have been shown to also significantly alter tendon stiffness over short time periods [13]. It would be of great interest to look at the impact other types of exercise have on the SWV in the AT in comparison to those found with running. Lastly, whilst the results of this study and other similar research [25] would indicate that the running-induced increase in AT stiffness is a temporary effect, other research does link long term adaptation of tendons to long term exercise training. There are currently no studies that trace the stiffness of an AT from sedentary to long term duration running, and none that have studied the AT stiffness of a long-term runner who stops training and therefore future research could elaborate on this.

In conclusion, this is the first study to utilise SWE to assess differences in leg dominance, trace the stiffness of the human AT in vivo during a normal working day and assess the impact of an acute bout of running. The results indicate that leg dominance does not affect SWE results in asymptomatic, healthy tendons, therefore the contra-lateral tendon may be used as a comparison for clinical investigation for this population. The time of day that a SWE measure is taken does not significantly alter AT stiffness and does not influence the measured values by more than 2.07%. Therefore, clinical appointments can be scheduled between 08:00 h and 17:00 h without affecting the measures taken, improving appointment accessibility when using SWE. Lastly, this study has shown that a 30-min run has no impact on AT length, however it does result in significant decreases in max AP diameter and significant increases in SWV measures, a surrogate measure of stiffness. The measured max AP diameter and SWV measures return to PRE-like values when measured 6 h after the exercise. This knowledge is vital to clinicians and researchers who will need to consider the presence of previous exercise when scanning with SWE as activity may potentially lead to misleading results.

Author Contributions: Conceptualization, C.P.; Data curation, C.P.; Formal analysis, C.P.; Investigation, C.P.; Methodology, C.P., P.W. and N.W.; Project administration, C.P.; Resources, C.P.; Software, C.P.; Supervision, P.W. and N.W.; Validation, C.P.; Visualization, C.P.; Writing-original draft, C.P.; Writing-review and editing, C.P., P.W. and N.W.

Funding: This research was supported by the University of Brighton who funded the studentship and purchased the necessary equipment.

Conflicts of Interest: The authors declare no conflict of interest.

References

1. Joseph, M.F.; Lillie, K.R.; Bergeron, D.J.; Deneqar, C.R. Measuring Achilles Tendon Mechanical Properties: A Reliable, Non-invasive method. *J. Strength Cond. Res.* **2012**, *26*, 2017–2020. [CrossRef] [PubMed]
2. Pearson, S.J.; Onambele, G.N.L. Influence of time of day on tendon compliance and estimations of voluntary activation levels. *Muscle Nerve* **2006**, *33*, 792–800. [CrossRef] [PubMed]
3. Onambele-Pearson, N.L.G.; Pearson, S.J. Time-of-day effect on patella tendon stiffness alters vastus lateralis fascicle length but not the quadriceps force-angle relationship. *J. Biomech.* **2007**, *40*, 1031–1037. [CrossRef] [PubMed]

4. Khan, K.M.; Scott, A. Mechanotherapy: How physical therapists' prescription of exercise promotes tissue repair. *Br. J. Sports Med.* **2009**, *43*, 247–252. [CrossRef] [PubMed]

5. Tuite, D.J.; Renström, P.A.F.H.; O'Brien, M. The aging tendon. *Scand. J. Med. Sci. Sports* **2007**, *7*, 72–77. [CrossRef]

6. Curwin, S. Rehabilitation after tendon injuries. In *Tendon Injuries: Basic Science and Clinical Medicine*; Maffulli, N., Renstrom, P., Leadbetter, W., Eds.; Springer International Publishing: London, UK, 2005; pp. 242–267.

7. Kjaer, M. Role of extracellular matrix in adaptation of tendon and skeletal muscle to mechanical loading. *Physiol. Rev.* **2004**, *84*, 649–698. [CrossRef] [PubMed]

8. Wang, J.H. Mechanobiology of tendon. *J. Biomech.* **2006**, *39*, 1563–1582. [CrossRef] [PubMed]

9. Magnusson, S.P.; Narici, M.V.; Maganaris, C.N.; Kiaer, M. Human tendon behaviour and adaptation, in vivo. *J. Physiol.* **2008**, *586*, 71–81. [CrossRef] [PubMed]

10. Obst, S.J.; Barrett, R.S.; Newsham-West, R. Immediate effect of exercise on achilles tendon properties: Systematic review. *Med. Sci. Sports Exerc.* **2013**, *45*, 1534–1544. [CrossRef] [PubMed]

11. Burgess, K.E.; Graham-smith, P.; Pearson, S.J. Effect of Acute Tensile Loading on Gender-Specific Tendon Structural and Mechanical Properties. *J. Orthop. Res.* **2009**, *27*, 510–516. [CrossRef] [PubMed]

12. Kato, E.; Kanehisa, H.; Fukunaga, T.; Kawakami, Y. Changes in ankle joint stiffness due to stretching: The role of tendon elongation of the gastrocnemius muscle. *Eur. J. Sport Sci.* **2010**, *10*, 111–119. [CrossRef]

13. Morse, C.I.; Degens, H.; Seynnes, O.R.; Maqanaris, C.N.; Jones, D.A. The acute effect of stretching on the passive stiffness of the human gastrocnemius muscle tendon unit. *J. Physiol.* **2008**, *586*, 97–106. [CrossRef] [PubMed]

14. Kubo, K.; Kanehisa, H.; Fukunaga, T. Effects of transient muscle contractions and stretching on the tendon structures in vivo. *Acta Physiol. Scand.* **2002**, *175*, 157–164. [CrossRef] [PubMed]

15. Kay, A.D.; Blazevich, A.J. Isometric contractions reduce plantar flexor moment, Achilles tendon stiffness, and neuromuscular activity but remove the subsequent effects of stretch. *J. Appl. Physiol.* **2009**, *107*, 1181–1189. [CrossRef] [PubMed]

16. Kay, A.D.; Blazevich, A.J. Concentric muscle contractions before static stretching minimize, but do not remove, stretch-induced force deficits. *J. Appl. Physiol.* **2010**, *108*, 637–645. [CrossRef] [PubMed]

17. Kubo, K.; Kanehisa, H.; Kawakami, Y.; Fukunaga, T. Influence of static stretching on viscoelastic properties of human tendon structures in vivo. *J. Appl. Physiol.* **2001**, *90*, 520–527. [CrossRef] [PubMed]

18. Nakamura, M.; Ikezoe, T.; Takeno, Y.; Ichihashi, N. Acute and prolonged effect of static stretching on the passive stiffness of the human gastrocnemius muscle tendon unit in vivo. *J. Orthop. Res.* **2011**, *29*, 1759–1763. [CrossRef] [PubMed]

19. Park, D.Y.; Rubenson, J.; Carr, A.; Mattson, J.; Besier, T.; Chou, L.B. Influence of Stretching and Warm-Up on Achilles Tendon Material Properties. *Foot Ankle Int.* **2011**, *32*, 407–413. [CrossRef] [PubMed]

20. Mademli, L.; Arampatzis, A.; Walsh, M. Effect of muscle fatigue on the compliance of the gastrocnemius medialis tendon and aponeurosis. *J. Biomech.* **2006**, *39*, 426–434. [CrossRef] [PubMed]

21. Mademli, L.; Arampatzis, A. Mechanical and morphological properties of the triceps surae muscle-tendon unit in old and young adults and their interaction with a submaximal fatiguing contraction. *J. Electromyogr. Kinesiol.* **2008**, *18*, 89–98. [CrossRef] [PubMed]

22. Mizuno, T.; Matsumoto, M.; Umemura, Y. Viscoelasticity of the muscle-tendon unit is returned more rapidly than range of motion after stretching. *Scand. J. Med. Sci. Sports* **2013**, *23*, 23–30. [CrossRef] [PubMed]

23. Farris, D.J.; Trewartha, G.; McGuigan, M.P. The effects of a 30-min run on the mechanics of the human Achilles tendon. *Eur. J. Appl. Physiol.* **2012**, *112*, 653–660. [CrossRef] [PubMed]

24. Peltonen, J.; Cronin, N.J.; Avela, J.; Finni, T. In vivo mechanical response of human Achilles tendon to a single bout of hopping exercise. *J. Exp. Biol.* **2010**, *213*, 1259–1265. [CrossRef] [PubMed]

25. Rosengarten, S.D.; Cook, J.L.; Bryant, A.L.; Cordy, J.T.; Daffy, J.; Docking, S.I. Australian football players' Achilles tendons respond to game loads within 2 days: An ultrasound tissue characterisation (UTC) study. *Br. J. Sports Med.* **2015**, *49*, 183–187. [CrossRef] [PubMed]

26. Kongsgaard, M.; Aagaard, P. Structural Achilles tendon properties in athletes subjected to different exercise modes and in Achilles tendon rupture patients. *J. Appl. Physiol.* **2005**, *99*, 1965–1971. [CrossRef] [PubMed]

27. Docking, S.I.; Cook, J. Pathological tendons maintain sufficient aligned fibrillar structure on ultrasound tissue characterization (UTC). *Scand. J. Med. Sci. Sports* **2015**, *26*, 1–9. [CrossRef] [PubMed]

28. Cook, J.L.; Purdam, C.R. Is tendon pathology a continuum? A pathology model to explain the clinical presentation of load-induced tendinopathy. *Br. J. Sports Med.* **2009**, *43*, 409–416. [CrossRef] [PubMed]

29. Hoskins, P.R. Principles of ultrasound elastography. *Ultrasound* **2012**, *20*, 8–15. [CrossRef]

30. Aubry, S.; Risson, J.; Kastler, A.; Barbier-Brion, B.; Siliman, G.; Runge, M.; Kastler, B. Biomechanical properties of the calcaneal tendon in vivo assessed by transient shear wave elastography. *Skelet. Radiol.* **2013**, *42*, 1143–1150. [CrossRef] [PubMed]

31. Arda, K.; Ciledag, N.; Aktas, E.; Aribas, B.K.; Köse, K. Quantitative assessment of normal soft-tissue elasticity using shear-wave ultrasound elastography. *AJR Am. J. Roentgenol.* **2011**, *197*, 532–536. [CrossRef] [PubMed]

32. Kot, B.C.W.; Zhang, Z.J.; Lee, A.W.C.; Leung, V.Y.; Fu, S.N. Elastic modulus of muscle and tendon with shear wave ultrasound elastography: Variations with different technical settings. *PLoS ONE* **2012**, *7*, e44348. [CrossRef] [PubMed]

33. Chen, X.; Cui, L.; He, P.; Shen, W.W.; Qian, Y.J.; Wang, J.R. Shear wave elastographic characterization of normal and torn achilles tendons a pilot study. *J. Ultrasound Med.* **2013**, *32*, 449–455. [CrossRef] [PubMed]

34. Peltz, C.D.; Haladik, J.A.; Divine, G.; Siegal, D.; van Holsbeeck, M.; Bey, M.J. ShearWave elastography: Repeatability for measurement of tendon stiffness. *Skelet. Radiol.* **2013**, *42*, 1151–1156. [CrossRef] [PubMed]

35. Miyamoto, N.; Hirata, K.; Kanehisa, H.; Yoshitake, Y. Validity of measurement of shear modulus by ultrasound shear wave elastography in human pennate muscle. *PLoS ONE* **2015**, *10*, e0124311. [CrossRef] [PubMed]

36. Eby, S.F.; Song, P.; Chen, S.; Chen, Q.; Greenleaf, J.F.; An, K.N. Validation of shear wave elastography in skeletal muscle. *J. Biomech.* **2013**, *46*, 2381–2387. [CrossRef] [PubMed]

37. Siu, W.; Chan, C.; Lam, C.; Lee, C.M.; Ying, M. Sonographic evaluation of the effect of long-term exercise on Achilles tendon stiffness using shear wave elastography. *J. Sci. Med. Sport* **2016**, *19*, 883–887. [CrossRef] [PubMed]

38. Pang, B.; Ying, M. Sonographic measurement of Achilles tendons in asymptomatic subjects. *J. Ultrasound Med.* **2006**, *25*, 1291–1296. [CrossRef] [PubMed]

39. Bohm, S.; Mersmann, F.; Marzilger, R.; Schroll, A.; Arampatzis, A. Asymmetry of Achilles tendon mechanical and morphological properties between both legs. *Scand. J. Med. Sci. Sports* **2015**, *25*, 124–132. [CrossRef] [PubMed]

40. Purcell, S.B.; Schuckman, B.E.; Docherty, C.L.; Schrader, J.; Poppy, W. Differences in ankle range of motion before and after exercise in 2 tape conditions. *Am. J. Sports Med.* **2009**, *37*, 383–389. [CrossRef] [PubMed]

41. Keles, S.B.; Sekir, U.; Gur, H.; Akova, B. Eccentric/concentric training of ankle evertor and dorsiflexors in recreational athletes: Muscle latency and strength. *Scand. J. Med. Sci. Sports* **2014**, *24*, e29–e38. [CrossRef] [PubMed]

42. Wu, Y.-K.; Lien, Y.-H.; Lin, K.-H.; Shih, T.T.; Wang, T.G.; Wang, H.K. Relationships between three potentiation effects of plyometric training and performance. *Scand. J. Med. Sci. Sports* **2010**, *20*, e80–e86. [CrossRef] [PubMed]

43. Borg, G. Psychophysical bases of perceived exertion. *Med. Sci. Sport Exerc.* **1982**, *14*, 377–381. [CrossRef]

44. Payne, C.; Webborn, N.; Watt, P.; Cercianani, M. Poor reproducibility of compression elastography in the Achilles tendon: Same day and consecutive day measurements. *Skelet. Radiol.* **2017**, *46*, 889–895. [CrossRef] [PubMed]

45. Beyer, R.; Kongsgaard, M.; Hougs Kjaer, B.; Øhlenschlæger, T.; Kjær, M.; Magnusson, S.P. Heavy Slow Resistance Versus Eccentric Training as Treatment for Achilles Tendinopathy: A Randomized Controlled Trial. *Am. J. Sports Med.* **2015**, *43*, 1704–1711. [CrossRef] [PubMed]

46. Ianculescu, V.; Ciolovan, L.M.; Dunant, A.; Vielh, P.; Mazouni, C.; Delaloge, S.; Dromain, C.; Blidaru, A.; Balleyguier, C. Added value of Virtual Touch IQ shear wave elastography in the ultrasound assessment of breast lesions. *Eur. J. Radiol.* **2014**, *83*, 773–777. [CrossRef] [PubMed]

47. Doherty, J.R.; Trahey, G.E.; Nightingale, K.R.; Palmeri, M.L. Acoustic radiation force elasticity imaging in diagnostic ultrasound. *IEEE Trans. Ultrason. Ferroelectr. Freq. Control* **2013**, *60*, 685–701. [CrossRef] [PubMed]

48. Gibbon, W.W.; Cooper, J.R.; Radcliffe, G.S. Sonographic incidence of tendon microtears in athletes with chronic Achilles tendinosis. *Br. J. Sports Med.* **1999**, *33*, 129–130. [CrossRef] [PubMed]

49. Docking, S.I.; Daffy, J.; van Schie, H.T.M.; Cook, J.L. Tendon structure changes after maximal exercise in the Thoroughbred horse: Use of ultrasound tissue characterisation to detect in vivo tendon response. *Vet. J.* **2012**, *194*, 338–342. [CrossRef] [PubMed]

50. Buchanan, C.I.; Marsh, R.L. Effects of exercise on the biomechanical, biochemical and structural properties of tendons. *Comp. Biochem. Physiol. A Mol. Integr. Physiol.* **2002**, *133*, 1101–1107. [CrossRef]

51. Leung, W.K.C.; Chu, K.L.; Lai, C. Sonographic evaluation of the immediate effects of eccentric heel drop exercise on Achilles tendon and gastrocnemius muscle stiffness using shear wave elastography. *Peer J.* **2017**, *5*, e3592. [CrossRef] [PubMed]

52. Chino, K.; Akagi, R.; Dohi, M.; Fukashiro, S.; Takahashi, H. Reliability and validity of quantifying absolute muscle hardness using ultrasound elastography. *PLoS ONE* **2012**, *7*, e45764. [CrossRef] [PubMed]

53. Brandenburg, J.E.; Eby, S.F.; Song, P.; Zhao, H.; Brault, J.S.; Chen, S.; An, K.N. Ultrasound elastography: The new frontier in direct measurement of muscle stiffness. *Arch. Phys. Med. Rehabil.* **2014**, *95*, 2207–2219. [CrossRef] [PubMed]

54. Payne, C.; Watt, P.; Cercignani, M.; Webborn, N. Reproducibility of shear wave elastography measures of the Achilles tendon. *Skelet. Radiol.* **2017**, *47*, 1–6. [CrossRef]

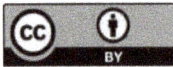

© 2018 by the authors. Licensee MDPI, Basel, Switzerland. This article is an open access article distributed under the terms and conditions of the Creative Commons Attribution (CC BY) license (http://creativecommons.org/licenses/by/4.0/).

*applied
sciences*

MDPI

Article

Strain Ratio as a Quantification Tool in Strain Imaging

Roald Flesland Havre [1,2,*], Jo Erling Riise Waage [3], Anesa Mulabecirovic [2,4],
Odd Helge Gilja [1,2,4] and Lars Birger Nesje [1,2,4]

[1] Department of Medicine, Haukeland University Hospital, 5021 Bergen, Norway; Odd.Gilja@uib.no (O.H.G.);
   Lars.Birger.Nesje@helse-bergen.no (L.B.N.)
[2] National Centre for Ultrasound in Gastroenterology, Haukeland University Hospital, 5021 Bergen, Norway;
   Anesa.Mulabecirovic@uib.no
[3] Department of Surgery, Nordsjællands Hospital, 3400 Hillerød, Denmark; jo.erling.riise.waage@regionh.dk
[4] Department of Clinical Medicine, University of Bergen, 5020 Bergen, Norway
* Correspondence: roald.flesland.havre@helse-bergen.no; Tel.: +47-55972872 or +47-90842938

Received: 22 June 2018; Accepted: 23 July 2018; Published: 1 August 2018

Featured Application: Strain-based elastography. In this paper, a Real-Time Elastography (Hitachi Medical Corporation, Zug, Switzerland) is used with relevant probes for external and endoscopic applications.

Abstract: Ultrasound-based strain imaging is available in several ultrasound (US) scanners. Strain ratio (SR) can be used to quantify the strain recorded simultaneously in two different user-selected areas, ideally exposed to the same amount of stress. The aim of this study was to evaluate SR variability when assessed in an in-vitro setup with a tissue-mimicking phantom on resected tissue samples and in live tissue scanning with endoscopic applications. We performed an in vivo retrospective analysis of SR variability used for quantification of elastic contrasts in a tissue-mimicking phantom containing four homogenous inclusion in 38 resected bowel wall lesions and 48 focal pancreatic lesions. Median SR and the inter-quartile range (IQR) were calculated for all external and endoscopic ultrasound (EUS) applications. The IQR and median provide a measure of SR variability focusing on the two percentiles of the data closest to the median value. The overall SR variability was lowest in a tissue-mimicking phantom (mean QR/median SR: 0.07). In resected bowel wall lesions representing adenomas, adenocarcinomas, or Crohn lesions, the variability increased (mean IQR/Median: 0.62). During an in vivo endoscopic examination of focal pancreatic lesions, the variability increased further (mean IQR/Median: 2.04). SR variability increased when assessed for different targets with growing heterogeneity and biological variability from homogeneous media to live tissues and endoscopic application. This may indicate a limitation for the accuracy of SR evaluation in some clinical applications.

Keywords: ultrasound; strain elastography; quantification; strain ratio; strain quantification; measurement variability; pancreas; endoscopic ultrasound (EUS); Crohn's disease; carcinoma

---

1. Introduction

Soft tissue elastic properties change in various pathological tissues, such as malignant tumors and inflammatory processes. Strain elastography can be used to quantify this physical feature based on ultrasound imaging. Tissue hardness can be assessed across tissue images describing the Elastic modulus (E), defined as the relationship between the application of local stress and the resulting strain. This can be expressed as:

$$E = \frac{\Delta \text{strain}}{\Delta \text{stress}} \tag{1}$$

Since the stress is not recorded as it travels from the stress source through the tissue as it gradually attenuates, calculating the Elastic modulus from strain data alone is not possible. This phenomenon is sometimes referred to as the "inverse problem" of strain elastography [1]. Under similar stress, strain in harder tissue is lower than strain in softer tissue [2,3]. Thus, a comparison between strain in the reference tissue and lesion produces a ratio that increases above one when the focal lesion is harder than the reference tissue. Strain ratio (*SR*) represents the relative difference in tissue hardness [4]. The definition of *SR* is:

$$Strain\ Ratio\ (SR) = \frac{Mean\ strain\ B\ (reference\ area)}{Mean\ strain\ A\ (lesion\ area)} \tag{2}$$

Hooke's law states that for small deformations in elastic media, the strain is linearly proportional with the force (stress) applied. However, this is true for isotropic and homogeneous media with near infinite or free border conditions. These conditions are rarely present in biological tissues, which exhibit non-linear elastic properties of different magnitudes due to differences in tissue structure and function. This may be of importance for the accuracy of strain elastography. By restricting the pre-compression and range of compressions (Δ-stress) to a limited interval, the stress–strain relation of the tissues involved may still be regarded as linear.

Vital tissue contains ducts and veins that act as stress dampers, as well as connective tissue and sliding anatomical surfaces that limit and enhance tissue movement, respectively. Unintended movements may cause strain concentration and reduce the accuracy of *SR* evaluation. Hence, in vivo conditions often do not meet the preconditions of Hooke´s law for elasticity calculation, and may therefore represent limitations and cause strain-imaging artefacts that increase variability and reduce the reproducibility of *SR* measurements.

SR expresses a momentarily and relative difference in compressibility in two user-selected areas within selected regions of interest in a strain elastogram. *SR* is dependent on similar stress applications in the two areas compared, and similar stress attenuation in the tissue between the stress source (probe) and the area of interest. The *SR* measurement method was first introduced as the "fat-lesion ratio" in breast imaging, where an area of subcutaneous fat was used as the reference to mean strain in the lesion under investigation. Using the subcutaneous fat as reference was perhaps as close to a standardized reference tissue as one can get. However, the same preconditions apply, as the tissue constitution between the probe and target lesion, and the probe distance may influence the strain distribution in reference area fat tissue.

The variations in elasticity of biological tissues is not linear with varying pre-compression or stretch of the tissue. For breast and pancreatic tissues, this has been evaluated by force indentation and deformation studies under increasing strength. This implies that the amount of pre-compression and the range of the stress applied influences the strain result and thereby the elastogram. In one study, the authors recommended a pre-compression level less than 0.2–0.4 kPa for breast imaging [5].

Another physical condition that complicates the reproducibility of strain ratios is the temporal variability in a live strain cine-loop. The best phases for acquiring strain data is during the compression and decompression phase, since no strain signal is transmitted when the stress is stable between these two phases. Compression and decompression of vital tissue may be caused by applied pressure from the probe or by natural internal movements from arterial pulsation, heart movements, or even breathing. Some strain elastography platforms provide feedback to the examiner about the phase of compression or decompression on which the image is acquired, enabling the use of *SR* from similar phases of tissue straining. One study on breast imaging concluded that peak *SR* performs better than average *SR* in breast tumor characterization [6].

Several studies reported high accuracy of *SR* in determining focal breast lesions as malignant or benign. In a meta-analysis, Sadigh et al. reported a sensitivity and a specificity of 88% and 83%, respectively, for *SR* with a receiver operating characteristic-area under curve (ROC-AUC) of 0.92. Strain elastography with *SR* has been compared to evaluation using a strain histogram with similar good results [7]. *SR* was reported to be better than magnetic resonance imaging (MRI) for breast tumor characterization, but the combination of the two modalities had a better ROC-AUC of 0.914 [8]. Furthermore, for the evaluation of axillary lymph nodes in breast cancer patients, a combined evaluation of B-mode ultrasound (US) and Real-Time Elastography (RTE) increased specificity [9]. Also, in the characterization of thyroid nodules as malignant or benign, *SR* was reported to have sensitivity of 85–89% with specificity of 80–82% in two meta-analyses [10,11]. In trans-rectal applications in prostate and rectal tumors, *SR* has been used to improve B-mode identification of malignant tumors with adequate accuracy (ROC-AUC > 90%) [12,13].

The aim of this study was to retrospectively compare variability in strain-based elastography quantified by *SR*, recorded in three different applications using Real-Time Elastography in homogeneous tissue-mimicking media, in resected tissue from bowel lesions, and during the endoscopic ultrasound (EUS) of focal pancreatic lesions. We chose to calculate the inter-quartile range (IQR) and median for all applications based on previous studies, since this has become a much-used quality-indicator in transient- and shear-wave elastography platforms. Our hypothesis is that *SR* measurement variability would increase substantially from phantom scanning to an endoscopic application on pancreatic lesions, which may limit the usefulness of the method in some applications.

2. Materials and Methods

The *SR* data in this study were recorded on the Hitachi (Hitachi Medical Corporation, Tokyo, Japan) Extended Combined Autocorrelation Method (ECAM) also known as Real-Time Elastography (RTE) operated on Hitachi HV-900 and Ascendus platforms (version: V16-04 STEP 2). US data were acquired using external linear probes (L54, 9–13 MHz). The phantom used was a standard model made of Zerdine® (US pat no. 5196343) embedded in a firm box including eight spherical inclusions with elasticities of 8, 14, 45, and 80 kPa in a background of 25 kPa (CIRS, model 49, Norfolk, Virginia, USA) (Figure 1).

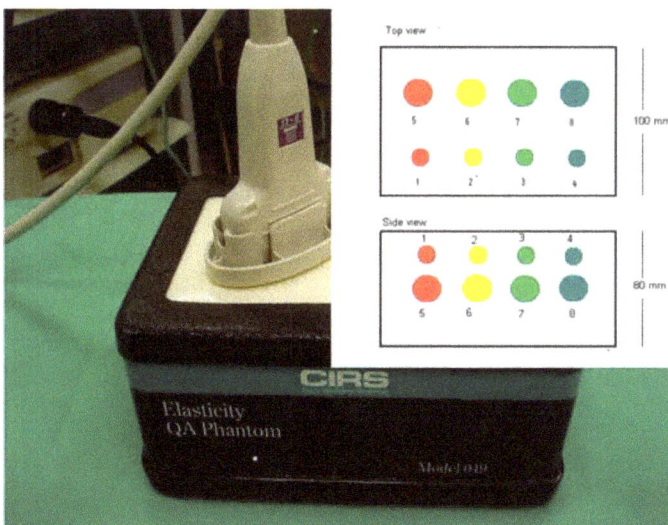

Figure 1. The Zerdine phantom used for scanning with a visualization of the inclusions inside. Red lesions: 8 kPa, yellow: 14 kPa, green: 45 kPa, and blue: 80 kPa in a background of 25 kPa.

To study surgical bowel specimens, we collected the specimens in the operation room, washed them, and proceeded directly to scanning in a designated scanning box with the bottom covered with 1 cm of agar. Bowel specimens were then fixated in formalin when attached to the bottom with colored pins, marking the scan-planes. A Hitachi HV-900 scanner was used with a L54 M linear probe, 9–13 MHz. We included 9 specimens from patients with Crohn's disease (16 sections scanned), 16 patients with adenocarcinomas (18 tumor sections scanned), and 3 patients with adenomas (4 lesion sections scanned). One patient had both an adenocarcinoma and an adenoma. Altogether, 38 sections of separate lesions were included. Histology was the reference standard. For further details on the patients and method, please refer to the original publication [14].

To examine pancreatic lesions, the data were recorded prospectively over a three-year period. We used Hitachi HV-900 with software version V16-04 STEP2. The echoendoscope was a Pentax EG-3870 UTK (Pentax Medical, Hamburg, Germany). We included 48 lesions from 39 patients: 11 adenocarcinomas, 7 malignant neuroendocrine tumors (NETs), 11 benign/indeterminate NET, 8 focal lesions in pancreatitis, 2 microcystic adenomas, and 9 other benign lesions. The reference standard was histology, EUS fine-needle-aspiration (FNA), or follow-up for at least 6 months. For further details and the diagnostic accuracy, please refer to the original publication [15].

Statistical Methods

We used the mean of the median *SR* values for each class of lesion, the range of values (max–min) and the interquartile range (IQR) for different objects or lesions. The IQR is a measure of the variability based on the two central quartiles from the 25th–75th percentile. The remaining 50% in the eccentric quartiles are not part of the IQR, but are accounted for by the range, representing the gap between the highest and lowest measured value. Kolmogorov–Smirnov's test was used to determine the distribution of data, and one-way Analysis of variance (ANOVA) or non-parametric tests were used accordingly. We then used the Kruskal–Wallis test for individual samples to compare the median *SR*, the IQR, and the IQR/median for the three applications of Real-Time Elastography with *SR*. We also analyzed the difference in median *SR*, IQR and IQR/median between observer A and B in the phantom and for benign or malignant pancreatic lesions by EUS elastography using one-way ANOVA and *t*-test. A difference with a *p*-value < 0.05 was considered statistically significant. We also used the intraclass correlation coefficient (ICC) to calculate inter observer agreement when possible.

All patients had signed a consent form to participate in the two studies that provided *SR* data for comparison of variability. For statistical analysis, we used SPSS, version 24 (SPSS, IBM, New York, NY, USA). Study protocols as well as patient information and consent forms were approved by the institutional committee for Research in Medicine and Biology. The studies were conducted according to the Helsinki Declaration for Research in Medicine and Biology. A excel file (Microsoft Corporation, Redmond, WA, USA) with the pooled data for phantom inclusions, surgical specimens and pancreatic lesions by entity is included as a Supplementary Materials file.

3. Results

In a homogeneous, tissue-mimicking phantom, four spherical inclusions with elasticity different from the background were examined by two different observers. Observer A had little experience with US scanning and observer B had extensive experience with both phantom and clinical application of US strain imaging methods. An image of inclusion 4 (80 ± 12 kPa) is shown in Figure 2.

In Table 1, the median values of 10 repeated *SR* measurements are reported for observer A and B, their range and interquartile range (IQR), and the IQR/median. The last measure represents the variability of 50% of the central observations divided by the median value. The common mean value for observers A and B was 0.07. The IQR for all median *SR* values for all inclusions was ≤0.17.

Table 1. Elastography strain ratio (*SR*) in four inclusions in a tissue-mimicking phantom.

Lesion Background 25 kPa	1 8 kPa		2 14 kPa		3 45 kPa		4 80 kPa	
Observer	A	B	A	B	A	B	A	B
Median *SR*	0.52	0.68	0.96	0.82	1.91	1.35	2.50	2.82
Range	0.09	0.08	1.04	0.10	0.18	0.11	0.91	0.24
IQR 1 25–75	0.06	0.03	0.15	0.06	0.12	0.04	0.17	0.07
IQR/Median	0.118	0.044	0.156	0.073	0.063	0.030	0.068	0.025

[1] IQR: Inter Quartile Range. Mean IQR/median for phantom lesions: 0.07.

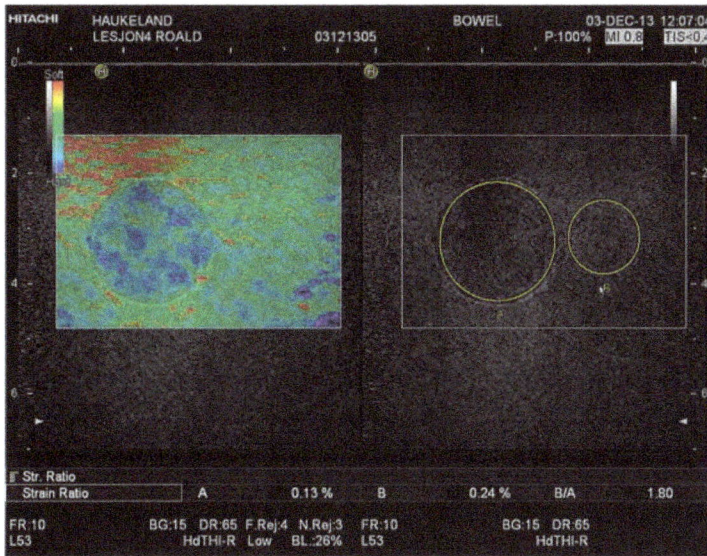

Figure 2. Elastogram from a tissue-mimicking phantom displaying a spherical inclusion (80 kPa) with a diameter of two cm in a background of 25 kPa. Right side: B-mode image with area markings. A (lesion) and B (reference). Left side: elastogram in color coding. The stress source was working from above in the axial direction. The lesion is speckled and green-blue, whereas the background material is mostly homogeneously green. Between the lesion and the probe, the red color indicates strain concentration between the stress source and the harder lesion. The strain ratio (*SR*) is mean strain in B/mean strain in A = 1.80.

3.1. Interobserver Variability

The interobserver variability in the phantom lesions expressed by the mean of the *SR* medians showed no significant difference between the two observers ($p = 0.937$ ANOVA). The IQR/median *SR* ranged from 0.063 to 0.156 (mean: 0.101) for observer A who had the least experience, and 0.025–0.073 (mean 0.043) for observer B who had more experience, but the difference was not significant ($p = 0.055$, ANOVA).

The distributions of median *SR* and IQR/median were not significantly different between observers A and B. The mean IQR alone was significantly different between observer A, at 0.125 (SD: 0.050), and observer B 0.050 (SD: 0.018) ($p = 0.027$ ANOVA). The range was not significantly different between the observers. The interobserver agreement assessed by intra-class correlation (ICC) for average measures between observer A and B was 0.661 ($p = 0.040$).

3.2. Strain Ratio in Surgical Specimens

One observer scanned surgically removed bowel specimens including tumors or resected Crohn lesions. The image of a scanned bowel wall with an adenocarcinoma is shown in Figure 3. The data on *SR* were previously published, but IQR/median was not used as a variability parameter [14]. *SR* was recorded between the normal bowel wall and peri-colic fat/connective tissue and the lesion of interest. *SR* results including range, IQR and IQR/median for the entities adenoma, Crohn lesions, and adenocarcinomas are reported in Table 2. Crohn lesions had a wide range in measurements (21.44), but they had the lowest IQR/median of 0.31. For adenocarcinomas, the IQR/median was 0.66 and for adenomas, represented by a limited number (4); the IQR/Median was 0.88. For all *SR* measurements of resected bowel tissue, the variability expressed by IQR was ≤0.88. The mean IQR/mean in all resected tissue was 0.62.

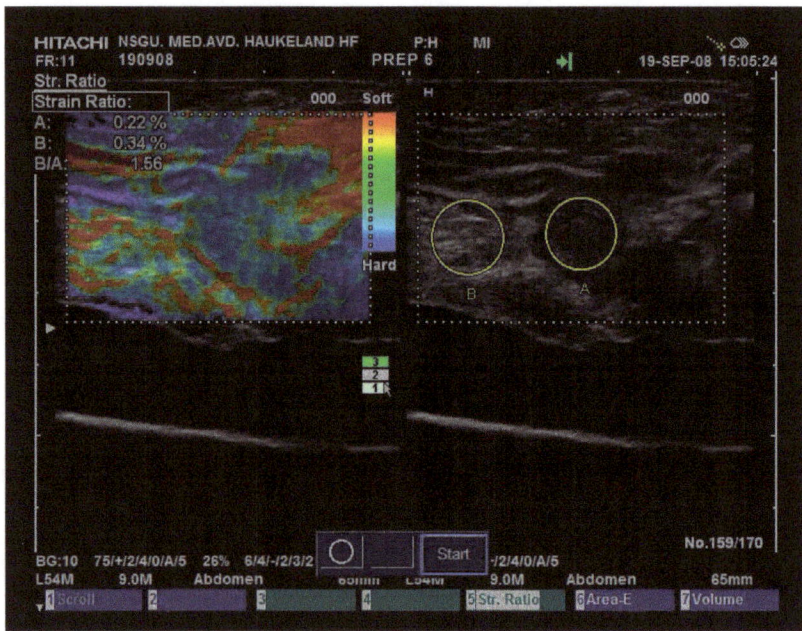

Figure 3. Elastogram of a newly resected bowel lesion from the colon containing a malignant tumor (adenocarcinoma). The hypoechoic tumor mass (**right**) is imaged with a blue-green color indicating harder tissue (**left**). The *SR* measured between pericolic fat and connective tissue, as well as part of the proper muscle and the tumor tissue, was 1.56. The lesion and reference are positioned at similar depth and distance from the stress source and the bottom.

Table 2. Elastography strain ratio (SR) in resected surgical bowel specimens.

Entity	Adenoma	Crohn	Adenocarcinoma
Number	4	16	18
Median *SR*	1.25	2.09	2.18
Range	1.38	21.44	4.53
IQR [1] (25–75)	1.10	0.64	1.44
IQR/Median	0.88	0.31	0.66

[1] IQR: Inter Quartile Range. Mean IQR/Median *SR* for ex vivo tissue: 0.62. Previously published in [14].

3.3. Strain Ratios in Live Tissue Using Endoscopic Ultrasound (EUS)

The data on pancreatic lesions representing various focal entities is reported in Table 3. The mean and range of these data had previously been published [15], but the IQR/median was not calculated and was not used as a variability parameter previously. The mean of median *SR* of the malignant pancreatic lesions was 7.05 (SD 1.85) and for the benign lesions, 2.15 (SD 1.22), ($p = 0.035$ *t*-test). For all entities, the IQR was higher than the median *SR* value, indicating substantial variability. For the malignant lesions the mean IQR/Median *SR* was 1.79 (SD 0.69) and for the benign lesions the mean IQR/Median *SR* was 2.21 (SD 1.29). The difference was not significant ($p = 0.713$, *t*-test). The mean IQR/Median *SR* for all pancreatic focal lesions by EUS elastography was 2.04. The IQR/Median SR value for lesions in focal pancreatitis was the highest (3.68), reflecting the large variability observed in focal pancreatitis as well as a relatively low median *SR* for this entity (0.91).

Table 3. Elastography strain ratio of focal pancreatic lesions by Endoscopic Ultrasound (EUS).

Entity	Neuroendocrine Tumors (NETs) Undetermined or Benign	NET Malignant	Adenocarcinoma	Focal Pancreatitis	Other Benign Lesion
Number	11	7	11	8	11
Median *SR*	2.19	5.74	8.36	0.91	3.34
Range	7.93	17.5	24.5	8.33	35.3
IQR [1] (25–75)	2.80	13.1	10.9	3.55	5.53
IQR/Median	1.28	2.28	1.30	3.68	1.66

[1] IQR: Inter Quartile Range. Mean IQR/Median *SR* for pancreatic lesions: 2.04. SR data with median values and IQR previously published as box-plots [15].

3.4. IQR/Median SR for Three Applications of Strain Elastography

For the three applications reported here, the IQR/median *SR* increased from scanning a tissue mimicking phantom to ex-vivo surgical specimens of bowel pathology, and increased further when the strain imaging was performed endoscopically focusing on focal pancreatic lesions. The difference between the IQR/median *SR* was significant ($p = 0.002$, Kruskal-Wallis; Figure 4).

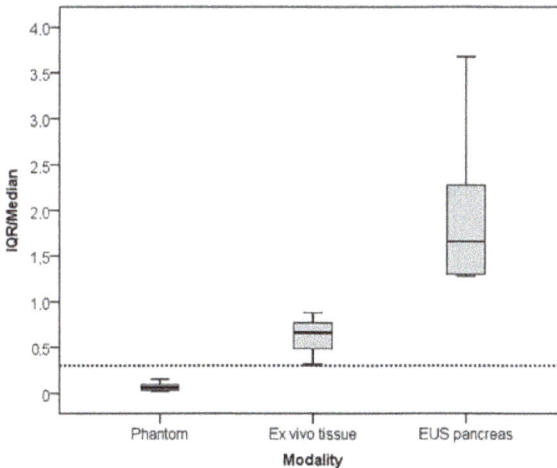

Figure 4. Box plots of the interquartile range (IQR)/median *SR* for the different applications of strain based elastography (Real-Time Elastography) reported here. There is significant difference between this quality parameter for the three applications ($p = 0.002$). In liver elastography using Transient Elastography, the suggested maximum IQR/Median Shear-Wave speed for good quality assessment in 10 repeated measurements in the same liver is 0.30, which is marked with the dotted horizontal line.

3.5. Reference Area Variability

Figure 5a–c demonstrate three different frames of strain images obtained with EUS elastography, including SR measurements of the same pancreatic tumor using slightly different but relevant reference areas. The three *SR*s obtained ranged from 8.43 to 16.36 to 25.70. All the variation was caused by variability in the reference tissue, in which strain varied between 0.08% to 0.16% to 0.27%. The lesion strain was 0.01% in all images.

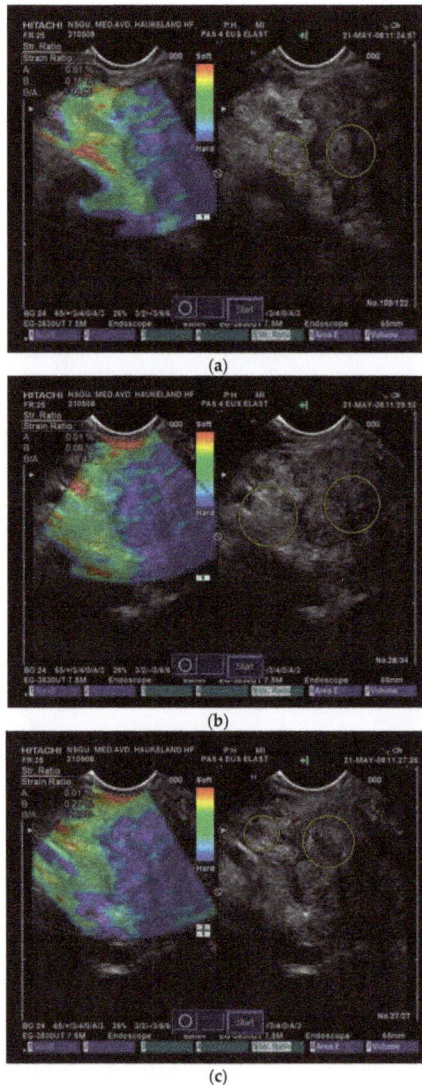

(a)

(b)

(c)

Figure 5. Three images of the same pancreatic tumor visualized by endoscopic ultrasound (EUS) elastography. Tumor tissue is blue in the elastograms with a predominantly green reference tissue. The position and size of the reference tissue vary slightly between the three different images, and exhibit different strains in all three images: (**a**) 0.16%; (**b**) 0.08%; and (**c**) 0.27%, whereas the strain in the lesion remained at 0.01%. This causes the *SR* values to vary from 8.43 to 26.7.

4. Discussion

In this paper, we presented *SR* measurement in a tissue-mimicking phantom and in resected tissue, where the stress was applied by pushing gently with the probe itself, focusing on the measurement variability. We also presented data from EUS elastography of focal pancreatic lesions where arterial pulsations, particularly from the aorta, acted as an internal stress source. We showed that the IQR increased with application to more complex anatomical structures and inability to control the stress source to a level that surpasses the median *SR* value. The mean value of the IQR/median increased 8.6 times from the phantom (0.07) to resected tissue (0.62) and 28.3 times with endosonographic application (2.04).

When applying strain elastography in an endoscopic application, the strain is dependent on endogenic stress sources, such as aortic pulsation and respiratory movements. These sources may vary considerably between patients and can hardly be standardized. Also, the availability of stable reference tissue that should be subject to similar stress as the lesion, may be hard to find in this application. Moreover, further differences may be caused by variable levels of pre-compression and applied stress caused by the endoscope. Since soft tissues have non-linear elastic properties, the tissue will appear harder with more applied stress or increased pre-compression [5,16]. An endoscopic application is also challenging because the probe is inserted into the gastrointestinal cavity and cannot be controlled directly by the observer's hands, as is the case with external strain imaging ultrasonography. Lu et al. performed a meta-analysis of EUS elastography in pancreatic lesions evaluated qualitatively with a visual score, strain histograms, *SR*, contrast enhanced EUS, and EUS FNA. They identified a large range in *SR* cut-off values based on previous published cut-off values or the ROC curves (3.05 to 24.82). This caused large heterogeneity for the specificity, and three-eighths of the studies were identified as outliers. After removing the outliers, the evaluation for identification of malignant lesions based on qualitative visual scores and strain histograms outperformed the *SR*-based evaluation (sensitivity: 0.94, specificity: 0.54, diagnostic odds ratio (OR): 29.42 [17]. However, strain elastography and *SR*-based assessment of rectal tumors using a dedicated radial rectal probe, which allows induction of strain by rapid water-inflation of a balloon around the US probe, was used to improve patient selection for organ-sparing treatment compared to standard multidisciplinary assessment [18].

In our experience, the variability in *SR* measurements increases when we transitioned from application with good access to relevant reference tissue, which allows for hand-eye coordination of inflicted stress, made possible by the real-time strain-feedback to the examiner on the screen. Selection of the reference area for comparison with a focal lesion also introduces variability that may influence the resulting *SR* more than the strain variability of the lesion itself, as illustrated in Figure 5. To avoid the variability induced by the reference area, some researchers recorded the strain values in the lesion of interest using the Strain Histogram (SH) function and found that it performed equally as well as the *SR* in some applications. However, this is dependent on a near standardized application of stress to the lesions of interest. The SH function displays the distribution of the different colors representing different strain intervals in a 256 scale, from no strain (0) to maximum strain (256), as set by the scanner software. From a histogram, quantifying the distribution of recorded strains it is also possible to evaluate if the lesion and reference tissue is homogeneous or heterogeneous by using kurtosis and range. Carlsen et al. showed that the SH (cut-off: 189) performed equally well as *SR* (cut-off: 1.44) in differentiating malignant from benign breast lesions, but the modality could not improve diagnostics when compared with radiological Breast Imaging-Reporting and Data System in a limited material [7]. The median value of the histogram represents the median hardness of the lesion. Opacic et al. suggested using the median histogram value of the reference tissue divided by the median value of the lesion histogram to create a histogram ratio. In a study of pancreatic lesions, this did not perform better than *SR* with a ROC-AUC of 0.843 and a cut-off selection yielding a specificity of 98%, a sensitivity of only 50%, and an accuracy of 69% [19]. Unfortunately, we did not record the strain histograms in our studies of surgical specimens and pancreatic lesions as this function was not available at the time.

Visual evaluation of the elastogram is direct and intuitive and requires no post-processing. Several scoring systems for categorical scoring of strain images have been proposed. For breast imaging, the five-point Tsukuba scale was proposed by Itoh et al. [20]. In two meta-analyses, *SR* measurements were found to differentiate malignant from benign breast lesions better than using the visual scoring range of one to five [21,22]. Amended versions of this visual score have been proposed for other organs, such as for the pancreas and lymph nodes by EUS elastography. Both the continuous visual analog scale (VAS) score and categorical visual scores for endoscopic assessment of rectal tumors has shown comparable results with *SR* measurements [23]. In a comparative study of *SR* and the five-point visual elastography breast scale, *SR* was more accurate. However, the direct visual impression of an experienced examiner using elastography imaging may contain more information than a five-step visual score can comprehend, which is useful in many cases for lesions in doubt. With training, different aspects of the elastogram, such as strain concentration and artefacts caused by veins and natural sliding surfaces, can be recognized. These findings can hardly be recognized by *SR*, histograms, or other formal quantification methods. One group investigated the use of automated pattern and color recognition of elastography of focal pancreatic lesions in 258 patients. They used an artificial neural network image analysis and information about the histological diagnosis from endoscopic elastography as the input. This improved the accuracy, with a ROC-AUC of 0.94, significantly better compared to using only lesion strain histograms that had a ROC-AUC of 0.85. This evaluation was performed using collected data in a multicenter study [24] but required substantial post-processing. In the future, automated tissue recognition or a material of standardized hardness, serving as a reference within the field-of-view, may be ways to improve *SR* in endoscopic applications. Also, averaging strain values over several frames or filtering noisy strain areas in the elastograms may improve *SR* measurements. We may possibly also soon see shear-wave elastography for flexible endoscopes.

Limitations

This study was based on previously recorded strain ratios from a tissue mimicking phantom and real tissues, both in vitro and in vivo. The data are based on different numbers of lesions for each application. For the resected tissue and the EUS elastography of pancreatic focal lesions, all recordings were performed by the same observer, whereas the phantom inclusions were performed by two observers. Because the data on surgical specimens and pancreatic lesions in this study were collected from individual lesions and patients, whereas the phantom inclusions represent only four different cases, this also limits the variability in the phantom *SR* measurements. The same strain elastography system was used for all scans (Hitachi, Real-Time Elastography), but both scanners and software were upgraded between the scanning of surgical specimens, EUS, and the phantom scanning. The ECAM algorithm was applied throughout all scans, but since elastograms are based on B-mode data, improvements in B-mode images through scanner software upgrades may have influenced the results. The scanning of the phantom was completed with the latest version of the scanner software.

5. Conclusions

SR measurements are useful for quantifying local differences in tissue strain and the evaluation method is well documented for several applications. We showed that *SR*, as a semi-quantitative method of strain elastography, has increasing variability when used in a tissue mimicking phantom, in resected surgical specimens, and for focal pancreatic lesions examined by endoscopic ultrasound. When the probe does not represent the source of stress or when a stable reference tissue cannot be obtained, *SR* may be subject to large variability and should be interpreted with caution.

Supplementary Materials: The following are available online at http://www.mdpi.com/2076-3417/8/8/1273/s1, Table 3, Pooled median *SR* values for phantom inclusions, surgical specimens and pancreatic focal lesions by diagnose.

Author Contributions: R.F.H. and L.B.N. and O.H.G. planned the studies and provided the equipment. L.B.N. and O.H.G. supervised in the collection of data, analyses and writing of the manuscript. R.F.H. collected and

Appl. Sci. **2018**, *8*, 1273

analyzed the data and wrote the manuscript. J.E.R.W. was a consultant in performing the elastography study on surgical specimens and pancreatic lesions with Real-Time Elastography. He also prepared the manuscript. A.M. participated in data collection and presented preliminary data at DDW 2016 as well as preparation of the manuscript.

Funding: This research was funded by the Department of Medicine, Haukeland University Hospital and University of Bergen, Institute of Clinical Medicine 1. These institutions provided salary and necessary equipment to perform the experiments described.

Acknowledgments: The studies that are reported data from in this paper were all conceived at the Department of Medicine and the National Centre for Ultrasound in Gastroenterology (NCGU), Haukeland University Hospital. We thank emeritus Svein Ødegaard for his tutoring and guidance and specialist nurse Eva Fosse for her great support during data acquisition. The studies were supported by MedViz, an interdisciplinary research cluster from Haukeland University Hospital, University of Bergen, and Christian Michelsen Research AS. We also express our gratitude to the support and guidance we have received from the application specialists in Hitachi Medical Corporation, Europe. Hitachi Medical Corporation has not provided equipment for free nor has had any influence on the planning, execution or reporting in the studies reported.

Conflicts of Interest: The authors declare no conflict of interest. The founding sponsors had no role in the design of the study; in the collection, analyses, or interpretation of data; in the writing of the manuscript, and in the decision to publish the results.

References

1. Aghajani, A.; Haghapanhi, M.; Nikazad, T. The Ultrasound Elastography Inverse Problem and the Effective Criteria. *Proc. Inst. Mech. Eng. H* **2013**, *11*, 1203–1212. [CrossRef] [PubMed]

2. Ophir, J.; Alam, S.K.; Garra, B.S.; Kallel, F.; Konofagou, E.E.; Krouskop, T.; Merritt, C.R.; Righetti, R.; Souchon, R.; Srinivasan, S.; et al. Elastography: Imaging the Elastic Properties of Soft Tissues with Ultrasound. *J. Med. Ultrason.* **2002**, *29*, 155. [CrossRef] [PubMed]

3. Ophir, J.; Cespedes, I.; Ponnekanti, H.; Yazdi, Y.; Li, X. Elastography: A Quantitative Method for Imaging the Elasticity of Biological Tissues. *Ultrason. Imaging* **1991**, *13*, 111–134. [CrossRef] [PubMed]

4. Ueno, E.; Umemoto, T.; Bando, H.; Tohno, E.; Waki, K.; Matsumura, T. New Quantitative Method in Breast Elastography: Fat Lesion Ratio (FLR). In Proceedings of the Radiological Society of North America Scientific Assembly and Annual Meeting, Chicago, IL, USA, 25–30 November 2007.

5. Umemoto, T.; Ueno, E.; Matsumura, T.; Yamakawa, M.; Bando, H.; Mitake, T.; Shiina, T. Ex Vivo and in Vivo Assessment of the Non-Linearity of Elasticity Properties of Breast Tissues for Quantitative Strain Elastography. *Ultrasound Med. Biol.* **2014**, *40*, 1755–1768. [CrossRef] [PubMed]

6. Le Sant, G.; Ates, F.; Brasseur, J.L.; Nordez, A. Elastography Study of Hamstring Behaviors During Passive Stretching. *PLoS ONE* **2015**, *10*. [CrossRef] [PubMed]

7. Carlsen, J.F.; Ewertsen, C.; Sletting, S.; Talman, M.L.; Vejborg, I.; Bachmann Nielsen, M. Strain Histograms are Equal to Strain Ratios in Predicting Malignancy in Breast Tumours. *PLoS ONE* **2017**, *12*. [CrossRef] [PubMed]

8. Cheng, R.; Li, J.; Ji, L.; Liu, H.; Zhu, L. Comparison of the Diagnostic Efficacy between Ultrasound Elastography and Magnetic Resonance Imaging for Breast Masses. *Exp. Ther. Med.* **2018**, *15*, 2519–2524. [CrossRef] [PubMed]

9. Xu, Y.; Bai, X.; Chen, Y.; Jiang, L.; Hu, B.; Hu, B.; Yu, L. Application of Real-Time Elastography Ultrasound in the Diagnosis of Axillary Lymph Node Metastasis in Breast Cancer Patients. *Sci. Rep.* **2018**, *8*, 10234. [CrossRef] [PubMed]

10. Razavi, S.A.; Hadduck, T.A.; Sadigh, G.; Dwamena, B.A. Comparative Effectiveness of Elastographic and B-Mode Ultrasound Criteria for Diagnostic Discrimination of Thyroid Nodules: A meta-analysis. *Am. J. Roentgenol.* **2013**, *200*, 1317–1326. [CrossRef] [PubMed]

11. Sun, J.; Cai, J.; Wang, X. Real-Time Ultrasound Elastography for Differentiation of Benign and Malignant Thyroid Nodules: A meta-analysis. *J. Ultrasound Med.* **2014**, *33*, 495–502. [CrossRef] [PubMed]

12. Waage, J.E.; Bach, S.P.; Pfeffer, F.; Leh, S.; Havre, R.F.; Odegaard, S.; Baatrup, G. Combined Endorectal Ultrasonography and Strain Elastography for the Staging of Early Rectal Cancer. *Colorectal Dis.* **2015**, *17*, 50–56. [CrossRef] [PubMed]

13. Zhang, Y.; Tang, J.; Li, Y.M.; Fei, X.; Lv, F.Q.; He, E.H.; Li, Q.Y.; Shi, H.Y. Differentiation of Prostate Cancer from Benign Lesions Using Strain Index of Transrectal Real-Time Tissue Elastography. *Eur. J. Radiol.* **2012**, *81*, 857–862. [CrossRef] [PubMed]

14. Havre, R.; Waage, J.E.; Leh, S.; Gilja, O.H.; Ødegaard, S.; Baatrup, G.; Nesje, L.B. Strain Assessment in Surgically Resected Inflammatory and Neoplastic Bowel Lesions. *Ultraschall Med.* **2014**, *35*, 149–158. [CrossRef] [PubMed]

15. Havre, R.F.; Odegaard, S.; Gilja, O.H.; Nesje, L.B. Characterization of Solid Focal Pancreatic Lesions Using Endoscopic Ultrasonography with Real-Time Elastography. *Scand. J. Gastroenterol.* **2014**, *49*, 742–751. [CrossRef] [PubMed]

16. Krouskop, T.A.; Wheeler, T.M.; Kallel, F.; Garra, B.S.; Hall, T. Elastic Moduli of Breast and Prostate Tissues under Compression. *Ultrason. Imaging* **1998**, *20*, 260–274. [CrossRef] [PubMed]

17. Lu, Y.; Chen, L.; Li, C.; Chen, H.; Chen, J. Diagnostic Utility of Endoscopic Ultrasonography-Elastography in the Evaluation of Solid Pancreatic Masses: A meta-analysis and systematic review. *Med. Ultrason.* **2017**, *19*, 150–158. [CrossRef] [PubMed]

18. Waage, J.E.; Leh, S.; Rosler, C.; Pfeffer, F.; Bach, S.P.; Havre, R.F.; Haldorsen, I.S.; Odegaard, S.; Baatrup, G. Endorectal Ultrasonography, Strain Elastography and MRI Differentiation of Rectal Adenomas and Adenocarcinomas. *Colorectal Dis.* **2015**, *17*, 124–131. [CrossRef] [PubMed]

19. Opacic, D.; Rustemovic, N.; Kalauz, M.; Markos, P.; Ostojic, Z.; Majerovic, M.; Ledinsky, I.; Visnjic, A.; Krznaric, J.; Opacic, M. Endoscopic Ultrasound Elastography Strain Histograms in the Evaluation of Patients with Pancreatic Masses. *World J. Gastroenterol.* **2015**, *21*, 4014–4019. [CrossRef] [PubMed]

20. Itoh, A.; Ueno, E.; Tohno, E.; Kamma, H.; Takahashi, H.; Shiina, T.; Yamakawa, M.; Matsumura, T. Breast Disease: Clinical Application of US Elastography for Diagnosis. *Radiology* **2006**, *239*, 341–350. [CrossRef] [PubMed]

21. Gong, X.; Xu, Q.; Xu, Z.; Xiong, P.; Yan, W.; Chen, Y. Real-Time Elastography for the Differentiation of Benign and Malignant Breast Lesions: A meta-analysis. *Breast Cancer Res. Treat.* **2011**, *130*, 11–18. [CrossRef] [PubMed]

22. Sadigh, G.; Carlos, R.C.; Neal, C.H.; Dwamena, B.A. Accuracy of Quantitative Ultrasound Elastography for Differentiation of Malignant and Benign Breast Abnormalities: A meta-analysis. *Breast Cancer Res. Treat.* **2012**, *134*, 923–931. [CrossRef] [PubMed]

23. Waage, J.E.; Rafaelsen, S.R.; Borley, N.R.; Havre, R.F.; Gubberud, E.T.; Leh, S.; Kolbro, T.; Hagen, K.K.; Eide, G.E.; Pfeffer, F. Strain Elastography Evaluation of Rectal Tumors: Inter- and intraobserver reproducibility. *Ultraschall Med.* **2015**, *36*, 611–617. [CrossRef] [PubMed]

24. Saftoiu, A.; Vilmann, P.; Gorunescu, F.; Janssen, J.; Hocke, M.; Larsen, M.; Iglesias-Garcia, J.; Arcidiacono, P.; Will, U.; Giovannini, M.; et al. Efficacy of an Artificial Neural Network-Based Approach to Endoscopic Ultrasound Elastography in Diagnosis of Focal Pancreatic Masses. *Clin. Gastroenterol. Hepatol.* **2012**, *10*, 84–90. [CrossRef] [PubMed]

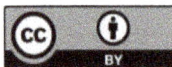

© 2018 by the authors. Licensee MDPI, Basel, Switzerland. This article is an open access article distributed under the terms and conditions of the Creative Commons Attribution (CC BY) license (http://creativecommons.org/licenses/by/4.0/).

MDPI

St. Alban-Anlage 66

4052 Basel

Switzerland

Tel. +41 61 683 77 34

Fax +41 61 302 89 18

www.mdpi.com

Applied Sciences Editorial Office

E-mail: applsci@mdpi.com

www.mdpi.com/journal/applsci

www.ingramcontent.com/pod-product-compliance
Lightning Source LLC
Chambersburg PA
CBHW051909210326
41597CB00033B/6080

* 9 7 8 3 0 3 8 9 7 9 1 0 4 *